MW01144375

ACE YOUR HEALTH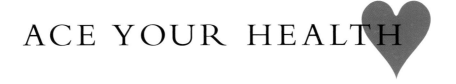

Please note that the page numbers listed in the contents and index are two higher than the actual pages of the book. The publisher apologizes for this inconvenience.

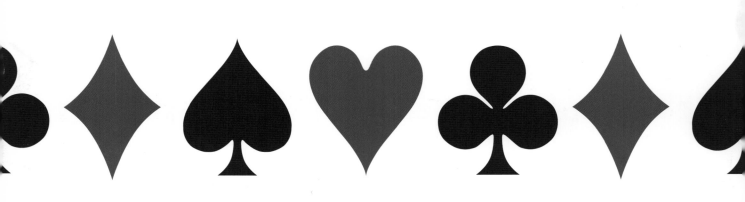

ACE YOUR HEALTH

52 WAYS TO STACK YOUR DECK

THERESA ALBERT

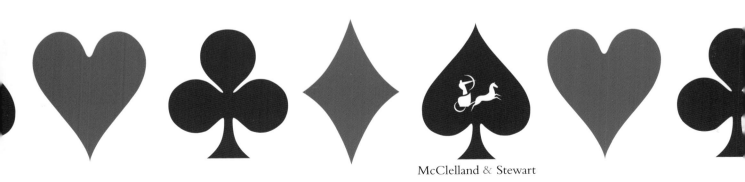

McClelland & Stewart

Copyright © 2011 by Theresa Albert

All rights reserved. The use of any part of this publication reproduced, transmitted in any form
or by any means, electronic, mechanical, photocopying, recording, or otherwise, or stored
in a retrieval system, without the prior written consent of the publisher – or, in case of photocopying
or other reprographic copying, a licence from the Canadian Copyright Licensing Agency – is an
infringement of the copyright law.

Library and Archives Canada Cataloguing in Publication

Albert, Theresa
    Ace your health : 52 ways to stack your deck / Theresa Albert.

Issued also in an electronic format.
ISBN 978-0-7710-0689-0

    1. Nutrition – Popular works. 2. Diet. 3. Health. I. Title.

RA784.A41 2010   613.2   C2010-903711-1

We acknowledge the financial support of the Government of Canada through the
Book Publishing Industry Development Program and that of the Government of Ontario
through the Ontario Media Development Corporation's Ontario Book Initiative.
We further acknowledge the support of the Canada Council for the Arts and the Ontario Arts Council
for our publishing program.

Published simultaneously in the United States of America by McClelland & Stewart Ltd.,
P.O. Box 1030, Plattsburgh, New York 12901

Library of Congress Control Number: 2010930256

Typeset in Bembo by M&S, Toronto
Printed and bound in China

McClelland & Stewart Ltd.
75 Sherbourne Street
Toronto, Ontario
M5A 2P9
www.mcclelland.com

1   2   3   4   5   15   14   13   12   11

For Guy and Jameson Ratchford.
I am honoured to be among you and feel privileged that you listen.
Thank you.

Contents

PART II ♥ | 83

WHAT YOU CAN DO TO KEEP IT PUMPING

PART III ♣ | 141

THE ANTI-AGING, ANTI-CANCER STUFF YOU JUST HAVE TO INCLUDE

PART IV ♦ | 199

LIFE'S HIDDEN GEMS AND WAYS TO FIT IN THE TIME TO ENJOY THEM

INTRODUCTION

Want to take a chance and play 52 Pick-up with your health? Didn't think so. And yet that is exactly what most of us are doing. We are stumbling from trend to trend, study to study, piecing together a system of living, eating, exercising, and being. What we need are a plan and a map to guide us through the often conflicting information on the news, in magazines, and on the shelves of the grocery store. With our fast-paced lives, it is no wonder more than 50 percent of us are overweight or obese, and that record numbers of people suffer from diabetes, heart attacks, strokes, and cancer. It is time to find a better way to live.

In life we are all dealt a hand to play. Some cards will be crappy genes, like the ones that put you at risk for major diseases like diabetes, cardiovascular disease, and cancer. But these conditions can all be prevented or managed with the right guidance. We just need a little training on how to take control of the hand and when to play or discard. With just a few shuffles in food, exercise, and health, those genes can, to a large degree, be turned on or off. After all, it's not whether you win or lose, it's how you play the game.

But who has time to read — let alone understand — all the nutritional news? One week we hear coffee is good for us, the next it's the worst thing we could put in our bodies! No wonder many of us have given up: who could blame us? What and whom should we believe?

Ace Your Health puts the whole game back in your hands. Its simple, practical approach walks you through your own life and shows you where you can make small changes for maximum benefit. *Ace Your Health* provides a once-a-week plan for you to make informed shifts in your thinking, your behaviour, your exercise, and your eating. Each week, you "play a card" and learn something new.

Each card is made up of three sections. First, I give you the whys and hows explained in a few hundred words, just enough to convince you but not enough to bore you. Then I pull it all together with a recipe. The recipes are as simple as they are delicious, and they use the ingredients or methods discussed in the chapter. After the recipe I give you a challenge so that you can practise your new knowledge, which helps the information stick. These challenges can be accommodated into any lifestyle. They are things you can do at the drive-through, restaurant, grocery store, or shopping mall. This fun system makes it easy to remember how to play the game for *life*.

How To Use This Book

My day job as a nutritionist in a preventative medicine facility gives me the opportunity to work with people who are motivated to become healthier but don't know where to start. I have structured the book with such people in mind. Designed like a deck of cards, *Ace Your Health* is ordered in suits. Within each suit, each card, from the Ace down to the Two represents a dietary or lifestyle change you can make. I explain that green tea is awesome but that its benefits won't save you if you are eating double bacon cheeseburgers every day. You have to start with the changes that make the most impact.

The suits are presented in a sequence − Spades, Hearts, Clubs, and Diamonds − and within each suit the cards are played in descending order (Aces are high) to ensure that the foundation is laid before the smaller (but still important) cards are played.

SPADES: These are the workhorses of the pack. They outline the big, difficult decisions that need to be made daily, such as:

- what to eat for breakfast to set your blood sugar level for sustained energy
- what to eat in a restaurant or food court that will enhance your health
- how to grocery shop quickly for maximum impact
- four things you need from the health food store (no matter how weird it smells in there)
- blockbuster healthy foods that are in your cupboard right now

HEARTS: I clarify what is truth and what is bunk when it comes to protecting your heart. At the end of this suit you will know:

- the truth about exercise (including how much is enough and how much is too much)
- how and why to get more and better sleep
- how often you can eat red meat and how to get away with it
- how to eat sauces without increasing your belt size

CLUBS: Often there is a socioeconomic divide in our approach to health. Those who have more money or education have more access to the "health club." You don't have to be able to afford a country club or a fitness club; everyone can join the *Ace Your Health* club of those who have crucial information. *Ace Your Health* gives you full access to all the secrets of better health.

The Clubs section shares:

- the secrets to anti-aging for your skin, body, and brain that don't cost an arm and a leg
- the fine line between enough and too much sunshine
- information on which foods fight cancer
- why a cast iron skillet is cheaper and better than a non-stick
- the differences between sugar and sweeteners

DIAMONDS: Diamonds are the gems that add sparkle to our lives; they represent the finer things we enjoy. Many of us need to focus more on the gems and less on being so darned perfect all the time. We need to slow down, but first we need to find out how:

- some supplements are crucial; others are crocks

- gentle stretching prevents injuries
- relaxing and sweating in a sauna helps clean your liver
- the difference between sounds and noise depends upon how you hear them

I strongly encourage you to do the challenges in each chapter; they are not hard and take little time. They are designed to help you engage with these new rules in the game of your life. If you want to "ace your health," you need to apply the principles in the challenges to your own life. I've seen the benefits first-hand. To help you stay on track, there are "Challenge Checklists" at the end of the book that relate to each suit. They will show you how to apply all the changes in a real day. You will be able to see what a great eating day looks like, using the recipes contained within each chapter. When you are finished each section, you have countless mix-and-match options to play with. There is also a Challenge Checklist that you can stick on the fridge or in some obvious place to remind you to act. Doing the challenges and checking off what you have done and learned is extremely motivating. Hey, if I could be in your kitchen each week coaxing you along, I would, but until then the Challenge Checklist will jog your memory.

Getting Started

The Lifestyle and Health Questionnaire at the beginning of the book is intended to encourage you to take a good hard look at what you know and how you are applying your current knowledge. It is designed to teach as well as to tease out your own truth, and operates on the premise that each of us must start from our own beginning and that none of us does everything right. We can all make improvements with more information, education, or perseverance.

Each suit builds upon the last, so each player will hit his or her stride at a different spot. The questionnaire provides a clue as to where that spot might be. No matter where you are in the game of your own health, you will find tips and tricks on how to play it better if you just follow the path I've laid out.

The book starts off assuming that you are average – blissfully, beautifully, average. You don't need to be anyone but who you are to get started. There is something for everyone that can be tweaked at any stage of the game. Read from the beginning, learn and implement the changes, and step it up where you think your game is lagging.

In every deck there is a spare card, in some games this card is wild, in others it is set aside. He is the joker and in this game you'll notice that he is missing. He is missing because I have assumed you won't need him as he has already been dealt out of your life. The Joker represents your decision to quit smoking. I haven't given him a place in the game because if you are still smoking, you have heard all you need to know to convince you to quit. Following the process of *Ace Your Health* will help you improve your health, but if you smoke you will always be playing catch-up. There is nothing that you can do from a health perspective that will overcome the damage you are doing by smoking. (This is the only depressing paragraph in the entire book. If he is still around I urge you to tear up your Joker as soon as you can.) Enough said.

As a chef and "greenie" I can't help but add: Depending upon *when* in the calendar year you start the process you may or may not be able to buy local. You should have as many fruits and vegetables as possible each and every day. If you can source locally and organically and stay with the program, I am beyond pleased. Next year, when all of the changes are old hat to you, you can adapt them to fit into your own seasons. Some foods (like avocado, kiwi, cocoa, tea) will never be available from local growers. They must be flown in from the tropics, but they are such great, versatile, and healthy foods that you need to include them in your diet.

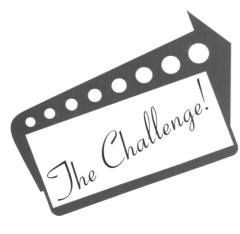

The Challenge!

IF YOU FOLLOW THE guidelines in *Ace Your Health*, excess weight will come off and you won't feel deprived. Your energy level will improve as your focus shifts and you learn more about your own life and body. You will move better (and your bowels will too), enjoy sugar and caffeine while avoiding the crashes, have a better chance at beating or preventing the onset of age-related diseases, breathe easier, and sleep like a baby.

By the end of the year, you will have taken a weekly lesson and played one kicker of a hand that will have had a positive impact on your life. You'll have developed your own game plan. You will be educated but without boring lectures, lies, New Age mumbo-jumbo, or scare tactics. You will never again be gambling with your own life once you *Ace Your Health*.

LIFESTYLE AND HEALTH

This quickie quiz will help determine where you are starting from on the healthy living continuum. It is designed as a fun way to illuminate a trend rather than give a score. Knowing which category you are in will help you know where to start and how quickly you can move through the levels of health. To gain insight, circle the statement that most closely reflects your behaviour. Don't worry if the answers aren't *exactly* as you would put them; it's your general attitude toward these decisions that matters. If two answers are close, circle both. And be honest; this is not a competition and you are the only player.

Ace: I eat a great breakfast daily.
- A: Yes! Never miss it and it contains protein as well as fibre.
- B: Yes! Never miss it.
- C: I skip it sometimes but usually have fruit.
- D: I either skip it or go for something at Starbucks or Tim's.

King: I exercise at least four times a week for at least 45 to 60 minutes.
- A: Of course, except for the week I take off to climb Mount Kilimanjaro.
- B: Well, more like three times a week for 30 to 45 minutes.
- C: I have a gym membership but don't get there often. I do try to walk a lot during the day, though.
- D: I can't seem to get this one right. I start an exercise regime but life keeps getting in the way.

Queen: I eat a healthy lunch every day of the week.
- A: Yes, and if I don't pack my own, I stick to vegetables and fish in restaurants.
- B: Most days, but occasionally I just can't resist a burger in the food court.
- C: I travel all of the time and am at the whim of clients, airports, take-out, or nothing at all.

D: Lunch? I never have time for lunch, are you kidding me?

Jack: Dinner is a pleasurable healthy experience that I enjoy before 8 p.m.

A: I make sure never to go to bed on a full stomach and eat at least three cups of vegetables at each dinner.

B: I do eat a healthy meal but it is often late and there is no avoiding that.

C: I eat late and lots because the day kind of gets away on me and I am starving by dinnertime.

D: I eat out a lot and sometimes dinner is rich and heavy.

10: I drink . . .

A: Alcohol on special occasions or not at all.

B: One or two glasses of wine two to five times a week.

C: Mostly wine and on most days.

D: I don't even want to answer, but I know it's more than I should.

9: I sleep . . .

A: Like a baby seven or eight hours a night without fail and without medication.

B: It's hard to get to sleep but once I get there, I am good for six to seven hours, which is enough.

C: I can get to sleep but I sleep lightly or wake up constantly and don't feel refreshed in the morning.

D: I don't need a lot of sleep but I feel tired in the afternoon.

8: I drink coffee . . .

A: Not at all or one cup every morning, but that's it.

B: Two or three cups a day but stop at noon.

C: Two or three cups a day, including one in the afternoon.

D: All day long, but it doesn't bother me.

7: I poop . . .

A: First thing in the morning before my coffee and sometimes once more during the day.

B: Once a day but usually after my coffee or tea.

C: Every other day but it's a good one.

D: Yeah, I kinda have a problem there, either too much or too little, too wet or too dry.

6: I drink water or herbal tea . . .

A: Two or three litres a day.

B: It varies but I am never thirsty.

C: I try to drink three or four glasses a day but I am constantly peeing!

D: Oh, gosh, I am a camel. Do I really need eight glasses?

5: My skin is . . .

A: Moist and supple.

B: Moist and supple, but I do get dry patches or rashes in the winter.

C: Fine if I use a lot of moisturizer.

D: I have acne or eczema.

4: My weight is . . .

A: Stable and I am happy with it.

B: Not my priority. I focus on being healthy, but if I lose a few pounds, that'd be good, too.

C: At least 20 pounds from being optimum.

D: My main preoccupation.

3: My salt intake is . . .

A: Under 2,000 milligrams per day, and I have tracked it.

B: Something that I ignore, but I don't use the salt shaker.

C: Not something that I think about often, but I know it's been in the news a lot lately.

D: Hard to control because I eat out a lot.

2: I eat loads of vegetables.

A: They are the foundation of every meal and I build the rest around it.

B: I love vegetables and eat six to eight servings per day.

C: I try to eat as many as I can but probably don't get enough.

D: There are only a few that I like.

Bonus wild card: I get enough of the right kind of protein.

A: I am vegetarian or vegan so I focus on getting at least four servings of tofu, nuts, hemp, and beans per day.

B: I get lots of tofu, nuts, hemp, and beans but also add fish, eggs, and chicken.

C: I eat all sorts of protein, mostly animal-based.

D: It just isn't a meal unless there is meat and I like a good steak two or three times a week.

Answer key:

This quiz gives an indication of where you are starting from, and there are better and less stellar answers that represent your choices. The food and lifestyle choices you make have a profound effect on your health. It is estimated that the age of onset or the very appearance of the most common age-related diseases (complications from obesity, heart disease, diabetes, cancer . . .) can be prolonged or prevented in 80 percent of the cases. This is largely due to our First World habits in diet and lifestyle alone. Count your circled answers and choose the category that fits you the best.

Mostly As

You are a Diamond player who has already figured out a lot of the right answers all on your own! Being someone who already does a lot of things right means that you just need to learn a few new plays. Doing so will tweak your game and help you eke every drop out of a healthy life.

Mostly Bs

Being in the Club category means that you are doing fairly well on your own. You probably read any news about nutrition and perhaps even subscribe to a health-oriented website or magazine. You are ready to step it up a bit to be sure that you are preventing diabetes, heart disease and cancer and are aging smartly.

Mostly Cs

You fall into the Hearts category. You are still working on your game and are interested in all the plays, but sometimes the rules conflict with your instincts. You try out every new idea that you hear about on the news or on *Oprah*, but not much sticks for long. The benefits of having a system to guide you are huge! Get in the game now and you will see changes very quickly.

Mostly Ds

You fall in to the Spades category. Kudos to you for even picking up this quiz! You have taken the first big step toward being in charge of your own health. Get ready to do some work and welcome to the game of life! Sticking with it will have a profound effect on your quality of life and put you back in control. Losing the weight and gaining the energy are easier than you think.

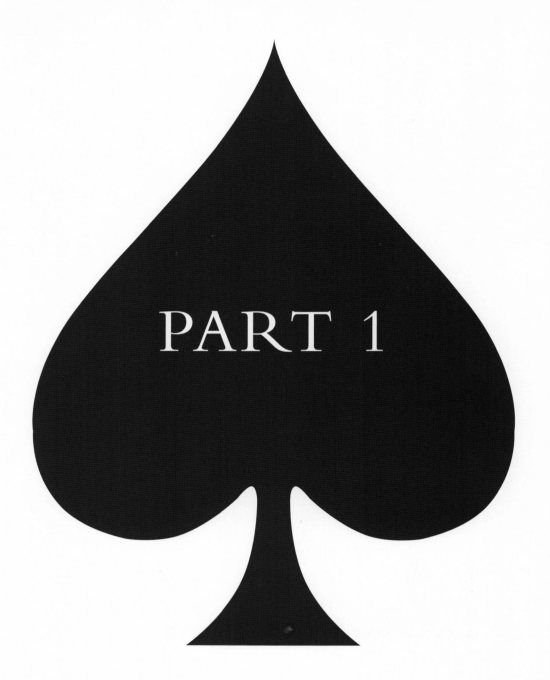

PART 1

*T*he cards in this section will have the biggest impact on how you feel right out of the gate. The overarching goal of this suit is to give you the tools to gain energy and to make good decisions toward your goal of living a healthier life. The places that you make many of these decisions are often not particularly healthy places; they're restaurants, food courts, and grocery stores. The better options are there but we often do not choose them in favour of savings and convenience.

But what if eating healthier didn't cost you more time or money? In fact, having just a touch of the crucial knowledge found in this section can save you both. And the bonus is better health, more energy, and a renewed vigour in taking an active role in your life.

For each card I'm giving you a tool that will help you change your eating habits for the better. Think of these changes as those that will make the first floor in a house of cards. Life is a house of cards, after all: tenuous and subject to all sorts of tragedy. And so the first step to a new and improved you is building a strong foundation based on knowledge and good choices.

ACE OF SPADES

BREAKFAST: Where it all starts

Breakfast is the most important play that you can make. I know you have heard this from your grandma on down, but if you are still not convinced, here are some things you should know. Study after study from respected researchers worldwide show that skipping breakfast is the single largest predictor of becoming overweight in adolescence, and overweight teenagers tend to become overweight adults. But this isn't the only reason you shouldn't skip breakfast. Having a meal within one hour of waking up keeps you from becoming sluggish in the afternoon, thus preventing the need to drink coffee late in the day – the very same coffee that will make you sleep fitfully, if at all, at night. That vicious cycle will ensure that your next day is less productive than the one before.

Your body wakes up and looks for a signal of what kind of day it will have. It wants to know what kind of food it will need to digest today and it responds accordingly. Like a Paleolithic hunter-gatherer, your body wants to know, Was the hunt successful? Can I count on you for protein or will we be gathering berries all day? If we are picking berries, I am going to need a lot of insulin to digest them and to get the most out of the fuel they have to offer. If I have protein, I may not have to work as hard. Your body thinks, "As I begin, so I will go," and behaves accordingly.

When your body gets lots of carbohydrates in the morning, it responds by giving you insulin to help with digestion. Sometimes your body will overshoot and create too much insulin, and the more often it does so, the more out of whack the process becomes. Too much insulin moves the fuel (in the form of glucose) from the blood to the cells, then stores it as fat! Your body thinks you are going to need fuel (fat) later because the large amount of energy (carbohydrates) you ate first thing signalled that you're packing it on in anticipation of a famine that is never going to come.

The good news is that each day's requirement is established anew. If you get enough protein at breakfast, along with fibre, your digestion will slow down and you will get a nice slow, gradual rise of insulin that will serve you throughout the day. Your body has now begun to trust that you have enough food to survive. This seems to be why eggs, which are a nutrient-rich and dense protein, are the best breakfast option (see Six of Clubs).

Setting a balanced blood sugar level in the morning makes the rest of the ride a little smoother. We all know that blood sugar spikes (like any highs) become crashes. If you avoid the spikes, you probably won't be "starving" by 11 a.m., and you won't be tempted to eat that doughnut during the morning meeting. Other-wise, you can't resist, your body won't let you; it's scared because it's crashing and sugar saves. Avoiding that crash is what having a protein-rich breakfast does. Your blood sugar will be stable enough not to drive you toward fast and furious calories. This early play sets up your next strategic play: a lunch that refuels you so that you can have a sensible snack at 3 p.m., instead of throw-ing the entire game for Ginny's birthday cake

and some java. It's all about giving you the tools in the morning when you have the courage to use them. Eating a proper breakfast gives you the strength to follow suit the rest of the day, naturally, with your biology co-operating.

But what else, other than eggs, can you have for a breakfast that is high in protein?

Here are three key foods: yogurt, hemp seeds, and white chia seeds. The last two may be new to you and I provide more explanation of these seeds in the King of Spades. Hemp seeds are almost pure protein at five grams per tablespoon and when they are combined with white chia seeds, which contain some protein and both soluble and insoluble fibre, you are set for the entire day! Yogurt is one of the few fermented foods that we eat and it is the fermented foods that lay the groundwork for a happy bowel. Remember the commercials with the Swiss guy yodelling his happiness long into his nineties because he ate yogurt? True story!

MAGIC MUESLI

You'll understand the magic by the third day, pinky swear!

Ingredients

		Benefits
½ cup	plain, low-fat yogurt	promotes bowel health
1	apple, grated*	phytonutrients
1 tbsp	uncooked oatmeal	lowers cholesterol
1 tbsp	slivered almonds	calcium and protein
1 tbsp	white chia seeds (see King of Spades)	high in fibre
½ cup	frozen blueberries	phenolics; enhance memory
¼ cup	hulled hemp seeds (see King of Spades)	protein; eco-friendly
1 tsp	ground cinnamon	lowers blood pressure
1 tsp	blackcurrant jam, to sweeten (optional)	urinary health

* or ½ cup unsweetened applesauce

Mix all the ingredients together and you will have the right amount of protein (about 10 grams), fibre, and nutrients to set you up for the day. Serve immediately or cover and keep in fridge up to 3 days.

Preparation time: **6 minutes** Servings: 2

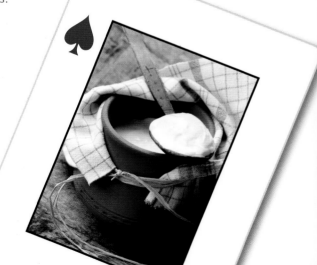

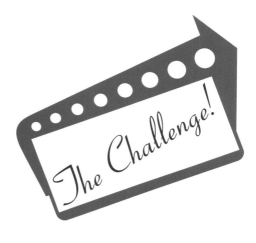

The Challenge!

THE FIRST WEEK'S GAME is played at the supermarket. Choosing a yogurt among the wide variety in the supermarket cooler is a feat in itself. Read the labels on three kinds: a plain, fat-free yogurt that does not contain any gelatin, a full-fat sweetened yogurt, and one with a cereal topper. Make sure the serving sizes are all the same. Now compare them in the chart.

TYPE OF YOGURT			
CALORIES			
FAT (g)			
SUGAR (g)			
PROTEIN (g)			
CALCIUM (%)			

By choosing a lower-fat, unsweetened yogurt over a sugary, full-fat one, you could cut out around 80 calories per day, which translates to a pound of weight loss in a month and a half. But calories are not the only factor. The range of added sugar can swing from 13 grams up to 22 grams, which has a direct impact on how much insulin your body needs to produce. To boot, higher-fat dairy products have more cholesterol, and if you can go with less in your yogurt, you may be able to enjoy something else that is more "worth it" later.

You can dress up plain yogurt with the ingredients in the Magic Muesli recipe and eat it for breakfast. Not only will you be ahead of the game, you will find it tastier than its sexy supermarket cousin.

KING OF SPADES

Avoiding health food stores is understandable. Let's face it, there are all kinds of weird things in there and the employees are intimidating experts on some pretty esoteric stuff. Plus, the stores smell funny! But once you get used to the smell, you'll see that they have lots of super-healthy foods. There is a perception that health food stores are expensive (which may not always be true), but there are also many online health food retailers, and I am a big fan of bulk food stores. And a lot of chain grocery stores have a small "natural foods" section that is worth dipping into.

The four health food items that are must-haves are hemp seeds, white chia seeds, nutritional (or "flaked") yeast, and miso paste. Rest assured, *Ace Your Health* isn't a book about a bunch of weird ingredients that you won't know how or when to use. These are the only few items and they are used in different ways and in various recipes throughout the deck.

Most health food stores are organized in sections. There is the body and bath section, the supplements, and the foods (sometimes these include produce). Frequently, there is a bulk section too and the following foods can be found either there or in the grains section, along with rice and pastas. Miso paste is sometimes refrigerated at the store, and you should definitely refrigerate it once it is opened.

HEMP SEEDS

These little nuggets are the best plant-source protein that money can buy. The reason you want plant sources of protein is because they tend to come in foods that contain only good fats (unlike steak) and that usually have more nutrients per calorie than animal sources. Hemp also has a symbiotic relationship with the planet, in that it actually puts nitrogen back into the soil (most other crops take nitrogen from the soil, which means they need to be fertilized, with compost in organic farming or with man-made fertilizers). Hemp also grows so vigorously that it does not need pesticides, so it's a true partner in sustainability. To boot, the stalks can be used as fibre for cloth and hemp oil is being developed as a biofuel. Hemp contains GLA (gamma-linolenic acid), which is a "good fat" (rarely found but vitally important in our diets), fibre, and liver-cleansing chlorophyll. Each tablespoon of hemp seeds contains five grams of protein, which is one-fifth what the average woman needs daily — that's a pretty powerful spoonful! These truly delicious seeds can be stirred into yogurt, sprinkled on salads, or topped onto vegetarian pizza to enhance flavour, texture, and nutritional content. Plus, they are the cheapest protein per nutrient available.

WHITE CHIA SEEDS

These tiny, crunchy, tasteless seeds (sometimes sold under the brand name Salba) are indeed the same type of seeds that grow on Chia Pets, but they are so much more. A favourite of Aztec warriors, these seeds have the most and best source of fibre around. Because they are perfectly round and swell evenly to absorb many, many times their weight in water, they are a smooth, gentle way of obtaining a "royal flush" of your bowels.

This grain is one of the few sources of plant-based omega-3 fats, which are crucial, anti-inflammatory fats. If that's not enough, these itty-bitty Peruvian powerhouses are ridiculously high in minerals and antioxidants that you aren't getting elsewhere. Chia seeds, like hemp seeds, can be sprinkled on everything. Buy the whole, unground seed. It doesn't need to be ground to be digested and you will be getting more bang for your buck. The ground version can become gummy, which works well in a smoothie or baked goods, but the whole seeds add a bit of texture and a cartload of additional minerals and vitamins.

NUTRITIONAL (OR FLAKED) YEAST

If you are old enough to recall the brewer's yeast health craze of the 1970s and '80s you may shudder at the thought of another bitter pill. But this version comes in a flaked form and can be added to savoury foods — and it tastes *waayy* better. Nutritional yeast is extremely high in B vitamins, the nutrients that (among many other things) help us to digest carbohydrates. The proper digestion of carbs is the secret of boundless energy. Simply put, more B vitamins equal more

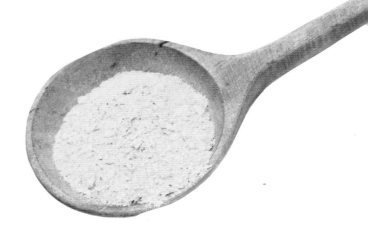

energy. Nutritional yeast tastes a little like Parmesan cheese. Stir it into any pasta sauce at the last possible second (it doesn't like heat) to add a creamy, cheesy element that is nutrient packed and unidentifiable. It adds a salty flavour without the salt – brilliant!

MISO PASTE

Fermented foods create a happy belly. The indigenous peoples of North America got their fermented elements from things like fish that had been buried for preservation, but our current diet doesn't have many sources. Thank goodness that immigrants have introduced us to their traditional foods. Miso paste is a versatile Japanese food. Yes, you have had it as miso soup in restaurants and this is a great way to start any meal, but you can do so much more with the paste. The paste is made from fermented soybeans and salt and it comes in various colours depending upon what else is in the mix, such as rice, barley, etc. White is the mildest, so it is a good place to start. A teaspoon stirred into any soup or stew (at the last second) is a great flavour and nutrient booster that will give your tummy what it needs to do its job effectively.

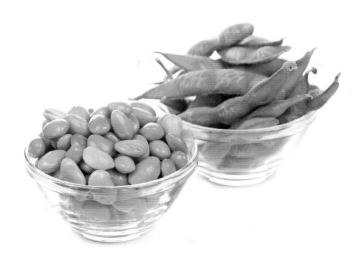

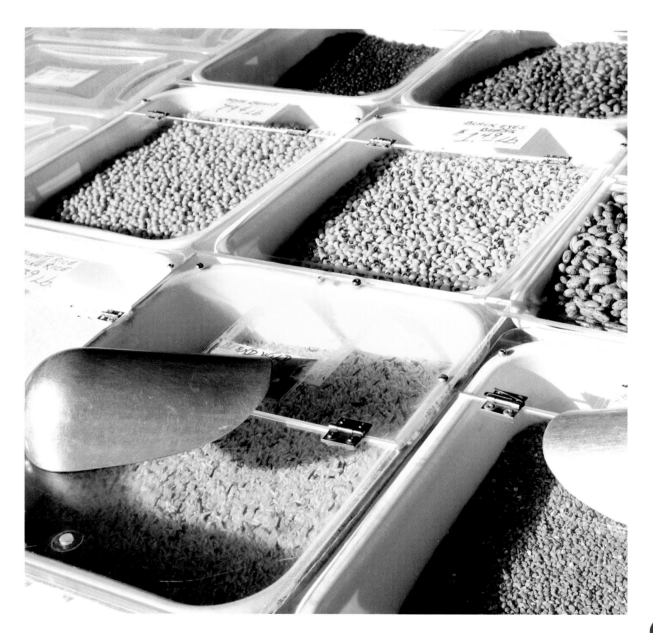

MISO DRESSING FOR SALADS AND FISH

Beyond soup, miso paste makes a delicious, versatile dressing that can be drizzled on salads and in marinades for fish. Gotta love this double-duty recipe!

	Ingredients	*Benefits*
¼ cup	grapeseed oil	improves cholesterol ratios
¼ cup	cold water	reduces salt per serving
2 tbsp	light miso paste	increases bowel efficiency
3 tbsp	rice vinegar (not "seasoned"), or white wine vinegar	helps alkalinity
1 tsp	cayenne pepper	boosts metabolism

Combine all ingredients in a glass jar. Dressing can be stored in the fridge for up to 2 weeks. Use to dress salads (2 tsp per person) or as a marinade for baked fish. Simply pour 2 teaspoons over 4–5 ounces of any white fish, then bake at 400°F for 10–15 minutes or until firm.

Preparation time: 15 seconds Servings: 24

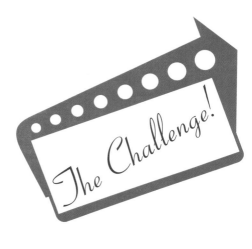

The Challenge!

GO TO A HEALTH food store when you have about a half-hour to spare. Take 15 minutes to stroll around, find the above four ingredients, plus one more item from the food shelf: something you know nothing about, a grain perhaps or a can of unfamiliar beans. Ask a staff member one question about this item, and see if he or she can suggest a recipe or a way to incorporate it into a meal. At home, look it up on the Internet and find new recipes to add to your personal collection.

Write about how you used the new food here:

_____

_____

_____

_____

_____

_____

_____

QUEEN OF SPADES

CAFFEINE: Coffee, tea – or energetic me?

_____

Is coffee your waker-upper or letter-downer? Do you have to give up your java to be healthy? Now that you know what to have for breakfast, let's clear up some confusion around the one thing that most of us really start our day with: coffee. The bottom line: If you are currently drinking coffee, you don't have to give it up; however, if you don't usually drink it, don't start!

Caffeine is a drug in that it stimulates the nervous system and has an addictive quality, but it has benefits, too. We each metabolize caffeine differently and some people have a higher tolerance. If you are one of the lucky few who is envied for her ability to have a big cup of coffee and go to bed 30 minutes later, read on and laugh. Realize, though, that the caffeine may be interfering with your sleep whether you feel it or not. The side effects of caffeine include muscle tremors, irregular heart rate, higher cholesterol, leaching of calcium from the bones, links to cancer, and reproductive effects like infertility and low birth rate. Plus, withdrawal can result in flu-like symptoms: headache, nausea, aches, and pains. Sometimes it is hard to pin down whether you are experiencing withdrawal or actual illness. If you have any doubt about

your caffeine intake and its relationship to your headaches, you will benefit from this week's challenge.

Health Canada recommends no more than 300 milligrams of caffeine for an adult woman daily; for men it is slightly more. That's three eight-ounce cups of coffee per day. The same amount of caffeine is found in about nine cups of black tea and 13 cups of green tea. There is also caffeine in pop and some pain medications, and you should account for that when tallying up your total caffeine intake. Until March 2010 manufacturers were allowed to add caffeine only to cola beverages in Canada, so we could be assured all other types of soda were caffeine-free. That decision has been changed and caffeine can be now added to any beverage. Health Canada still suggests that we consume no more than the recommended amount of caffeine but gives us and our kids more places to find it.

As more research is conducted on the effects of caffeine, the picture is becoming clearer and the news is not all bad. Turns out that there are some health benefits to drinking coffee and tea. Here is my dividing line: if there are other, natural nutrients in your source of caffeine (as in coffee and tea), it can stay; if it is added to something that contains sugar, corn sweeteners, and/or colouring, dump it.

Coffee has been studied for its positive effects not only on alertness (we all know how it can help you get through a long drive or a boring boardroom meeting), but also on reducing the risk of some diseases. One to three cups of coffee per day can reduce the risk of diabetes, Parkinson's, colon cancer, cirrhosis of the liver, and gallstones. It is still not clear exactly what in coffee has an impact, but we do know that caffeine does play a role because decaf did not perform as well in tests. The antioxidants in the beans themselves, as well as their antibacterial properties, can't be ruled out. In short, your moderate intake of coffee can stay.

Tea is even higher in health-preserving antioxidants and shows the same kind of promise, but it is lower in caffeine and the differential makes tea a healthier choice — more of the good stuff and less of the bad (addictive) stuff. Most of us drink orange pekoe or Earl Grey, which would be considered black tea, which is exactly the same leaf as green tea only it has been fermented. Black teas are good as long as you drink them clear; the protein in milk appears to block the uptake of the antioxidants. Green tea seems to retain more of its antioxidant strength and is slightly lower in caffeine, so you can drink more of it for your caffeine quota (which also increases your daily water intake).

So, if you are a five-cup-per-day coffee drinker (and even the "small" coffee shop cup can contain 12 ounces of coffee, never mind the large, which can be up to 24 ounces!), you should reduce your consumption to a maximum of three eight-ounce cups per day. If you can get down to the maximums listed below and stay there, you have accomplished what we set out to do (if you go lower, you are ahead of the game).

- a maximum of eight ounces of your favourite coffee in the morning
- a maximum of eight ounces of orange pekoe or any other black tea (clear or with honey) at 10 a.m.
- up to 16 ounces of green tea in the afternoon, stopping by 3 p.m.

Of course, you will want to take baby steps toward this goal. It is highly improbable that you can jump from your five cups of coffee a day down to one overnight. You will hate (and likely throw away) this book in a fit of anger induced by headache and irritability. We want a slow shift, not an earthquake, so cut back on the coffee one-half cup at a time. Start with your last one in the day and move backward to drinking it to 3 p.m., at the latest. It's best to have completely caffeine-free afternoons, which will help you to sleep better, but, if life's too short for you to be that perfect, 3 p.m. works. For a delicious coffee-like beverage that is completely caffeine-free, try the following recipe.

ICED MAPLE CAPPUCCINO

It is possible to have a caffeine-free coffee-like beverage that is a heavenly, low–cal treat! Roasted chicory coffee substitute is an instant grain that tastes remarkably like coffee but has zero caffeine (unlike decaf, which has traces). That means you don't have to count it in your total. Roasted chicory is commonly found in any grocery store in the coffee aisle. It was big during the Second World War when coffee was scarce – your mother or grandmother will know all about it!

	Ingredients	*Benefits*
2 tbsp	boiling water	cleanses the liver
1 tbsp	roasted chicory coffee substitute	contains prebiotics
2 tsp	maple syrup	zinc; promotes clear skin
2¼ cups	1% low-fat milk	multi-minerals, including calcium
6	ice cubes	zero-calorie froth
pinch	ground cinnamon	lowers blood pressure

In a blender, combine boiling water, chicory, and maple syrup. Blend for 20 seconds. Add milk and ice cubes, blend until ice is crushed. Pour into 2 glasses and top with cinnamon.

Preparation time: 3 minutes Servings: 2

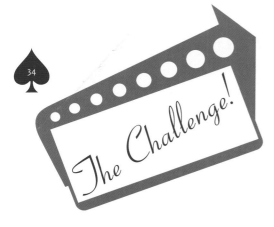

The Challenge!

DRINK EXACTLY THE SAME measured brew at exactly the same time each day for three days and make a note of how much and what time you had your coffee or tea. If you do not get a headache that week, you are now a well-controlled addict. Each day for the rest of the week, drop one half-cup from your routine and see if you have symptoms of headache or fogginess. This whole process could take longer than a week. Try switching your later-in-the-day coffees to black tea and then green tea. I'll catch up with you in the Three of Hearts (Tea) and amp your game up even further.

Record all sources and amounts of caffeine in a typical day. Don't forget to read all beverage labels, and check labels and/or with a pharmacist about any drugs you take that may contain caffeine, especially pain and migraine medications.

CAFFEINE SOURCE	TIME OF DAY	AMOUNT (mg)	MOOD/ENERGY HEADACHE/SLEEP SYMPTOMS
DAY 1			
DAY 2			
DAY 3			
DAY 4			
DAY 5			
DAY 6			
DAY 7			

JACK OF SPADES

FOOD COURTS: Courting a nourishing lunch

Whether you are working at a desk all day or digging up concrete, your body is burning energy all the while. The brain needs fuel to keep coming up with those brilliant ideas just as much as the biceps need it to move. Mind you, they are different needs: the brain needs more nutrients while the biceps need more calories. But still, whatever your situation, it's best to take food breaks and give your body what it requires to keep you going.

In a *perfect world*, you would pack lunches that come from last night's dinner. You would think ahead and bake an extra chicken breast or two to chop into a massive container of salad. Your lunch would also contain a whole piece of fruit with the skin on and a large container of water. Four whole-grain crackers or flatbreads would keep the carbohydrates in check. A container of yogurt for dessert would round out the food groups.

In the *real world*, if we remember to pack a lunch at all, usually it's carbohydrate heavy. Folklore tells us that the sandwich, our most common lunch item, was invented so that the Earl of Sandwich wouldn't have to interrupt his card game to eat. He could keep playing and consume as many calories as possible with one hand! That isn't exactly what we modern folks want from this meal.

So, what if you forgot or were too busy to prepare a lunch and are now faced with foraging at the food court? Food courts *have* improved over the years and the fryer no longer holds sole sway. A food court can be a fine place to eat a maximum of two days per week, as long as you follow my Number One Rule: nothing deep-fried.

You need to choose menu items that contain more protein and vegetables than carbohydrates. That rules out almost anything on bread or a bun: they are simply too high in the kind of fuel (carbs) that burns up quickly and pushes you smack into a 3 p.m. crash. However, if you are doing physical labour, have the bread, because you will burn that fuel. Just make sure it is whole-grain.

Eliminating bread can mean choosing Asian dishes, but don't fall into the white-rice trap, which is right next to the deep-fried ambush (chicken balls and crispy beef dishes: *crispy* is code for deep-fried). Look for veggies and protein in a stir fry. You will be surprised by how much stir-fried broccoli you can eat for the same number of calories as is in white rice. Don't just think Chinese! Go Thai — even with the coconut sauce, as long as you skip the rice. Go Japanese — teriyaki salmon, chicken, or beef, even sushi as long as it's made with brown rice.

The trick is in the chewing. It is virtually impossible to wolf down chunky meat and veggies the way you can a soft, supple sandwich or bowl of pasta. These soft foods are "comfort foods" for a reason; they offer instant gratification. The brain hardly has time to register the intake of food before the pancreas, whose job it is to regulate insulin, kicks into overdrive. Less chewing and high insulin means that messages signalling you're full don't reach the brain quickly enough. Your brain and your pancreas are in collusion, trying to keep you energized and satisfied, and we want them working together, not squabbling over whether you have eaten enough, or whether you are burning or conserving calories. You can help them make peace by eating fibre- and nutrient-dense foods.

ALMOND CHICKEN

Lunch planning is simple when you bake a bunch of chicken breasts at the beginning of the week. Wrap in single-serving packages and you are golden. This recipe is for easy, tasty, crispy baked breasts. Scale up the recipe to accommodate the number of people in your household.

Ingredients / *Benefits*

4	boneless, skinless chicken breast halves	lean protein; repairs DNA
½ cup	ground almonds	calcium for bones
1 tbsp	Dijon mustard	low- cal, high-flavour
2 tbsp	cornmeal	fibre for healthy bowels
	white wine or water, to thin	
1 tsp	dill seed	phytonutrients; fight free radicals
3 tbsp	balsamic vinegar	resveratrol for heart health

Lay breasts on a cookie sheet that has been sprayed with cooking oil. Mix remaining ingredients together, using just enough wine or water to make a paste about as thick as mustard. Divide paste among breasts, and smear evenly. Cover with foil. Bake in 350°F oven, 45–55 minutes (to an internal temperature of 165°F) depending on thickness of breasts. Remove foil about halfway through cooking. Cool and store in fridge up to 4 days or in freezer up to 2 weeks. Serve for lunches with salad greens or veggies and dip.

Preparation time: 5 minutes Servings: 4

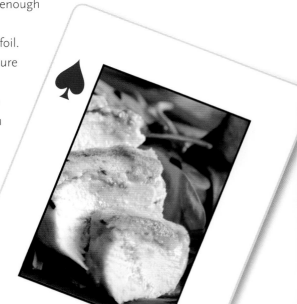

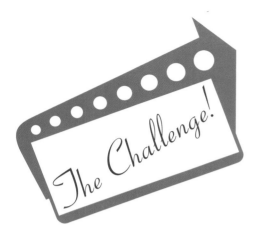

The Challenge!

YOUR CHALLENGE THIS WEEK is to uncover your food court options. You are looking for the meal that has at least 8 grams of fibre (you need to get over 25 every day) and 10 grams of protein (you need between 40 and 75 grams, depending upon gender and size) while providing no more than 350 to 600 calories. A wide range of calories, but the other two numbers are more important, and the calories required really depend upon the rest of the food in your day and your activity level.

Ask as many outlets as possible for their nutritional information handouts. Once you have these in hand, write down your three favourite meals below, ensuring that the serving size quoted is what is actually served – these numbers can be sneaky! Keep in mind that our absolute maximum intake of sodium is between 2,000 and 2,500 milligrams per day (many experts think that this is double what it should be), so you may have to make up elsewhere in your day for the excess salt you will be eating (see Seven of Hearts).

FOOD COURT OUTLET	FAVOURITE DISHES	SERVING SIZE	SODIUM (g)

TEN OF SPADES

DINING OUT: Restaurant survival plays

Those of us who dine out once a month or less need to be as smart as we can when choosing our meals, and then make up for it the next day with an extra mile on the treadmill and a tighter hold on the reins. (You need to work off an extra 200 to 500 calories for every restaurant meal you indulge in.) But many people are in situations where they have to eat out more often. In my practice I see a lot of people who have a hard time maintaining portion control and, therefore, weight because they frequently have to eat in restaurants. Sometimes it's because they travel or entertain, but often it's just the speed of life.

With large portion sizes and the liberal use of butter, oils, and other fats, restaurant meals can mean an extra 200 calories per meal. If we extend that over three meals per day, five days per week, it can add up to a pound gained per week. Jet-setters need to either compensate on the weekends or learn how to eat well despite their lifestyle. Luckily, we can all learn from their lessons.

One strategy is to make your weekends no-resto zones. If weekends are lean and mean and veggie-packed affairs without caloric alcohol, you might just maintain an even keel. It's easier, though, to learn how to manage to get enough nutrients, fewer calories, and leaner eats on the go. Then you can still have some fun on the weekends.

RESTO RULES

Offer to choose the restaurant for the party and make the reservation. This will allow you to be sure there is something tasty that you can eat. Buffets are the very last resort: too many bad choices equals too much temptation.

The best choices are:
- Asian (only sushi made with brown rice); stir-fried, grilled, or teriyaki chicken or fish (see Jack of Hearts)
- Greek (grilled meats and veg, go easy on the dips)
- Other Mediterranean
- Seafood or shellfish, grilled
- Contemporary fresh (vegetarian, vegan, raw . . .)

Whatever kind of resto you eat at, here are some tips on ordering:

- Send away the bread basket if your tablemates agree (you can ask for it back later when you are full of good, worthwhile food).
- Ask for a large glass of ice water and drink it all before you eat anything.
- Decide how many alcoholic drinks you will have now (before you have two and your defences go down and you tell yourself: "Oh, c'mon, one more won't make that much difference." It will!) Avoid mixed drinks and sugary soft drinks (see Eight of Diamonds). Have one wine or beer or one shot of alcohol with soda and lime.
- Order a broth or puréed vegetable soup (no cream); this is even better than a salad (see Six of Hearts).
- If you have a salad, order the dressing on the side and ask for fresh lemon. A teaspoon of dressing goes much further watered down with zippy lemon. No croutons!
- Ask for a takeout container right away and put half your meal into it. If you are eco-keen, carry a reusable container with you.
- In descending order, choices should be: fish, chicken, pork tenderloin, lamb chops, beef tenderloin (all animal proteins should be broiled or grilled).
- If you can, skip the starchy side dishes. If not, choose in the following order: baked sweet or white potato, soba noodles, brown rice (only!). If fries are your only option or your first love, choose sweet potato fries and have exactly 10.
- Order double of your vegetable dishes. Go for steamed. Choose green. Ask for no butter or oil.
- If you have pasta as a main course, ask for twice the tomato sauce and veggies and half the pasta. (You may be asked to pay an extra dollar or two, but you won't have to spend the extra 30 minutes on the treadmill.) Ask for whole-wheat noodles. No oil- or cream-based sauces.
- Choose spicy dishes and/or add black pepper. Hot seasonings increase your metabolism ever so slightly and will help you burn calories.
- For dessert, share or have three bites of anything you want, but only once a week (see Four of Diamonds).

If you are used to having a hot beverage after your meal, make sure it is as low-cal as possible. Mint tea hits the spot, as does a steamed skim milk or decaf espresso. No cream and no sugar. (Having a hot drink at the end of a meal sends a satiety signal to your brain that it is time to stop eating.)

ROOM SERVICE BANANA OATMEAL

Breakfast on the road can be just as fraught as lunch or dinner. This recipe works well at home but is portable for the road. When you travel, always carry with you two of the health food store items that you purchased with the King of Spades: white chia and hemp (both travel well in little zipper baggies). I have many clients and colleagues who travel with their own breakfast in a bag.

Order hot oatmeal, a fork and a banana from room service. Ask for real maple syrup, too, which goes a lot further in flavour than brown sugar. Make sure you get the syrup on the side. Double-check that the restaurant cooks your oats in water, not cream! The more stars the establishment sports the more likely it uses cream. If you like cream on your oatmeal, work your way gradually toward skim milk, reducing from 35 percent or 18 percent fat, and so on, to zero. (Money-saving tip: Travel with little packets of plain, unsweetened, unsalted instant oats. Ask for a kettle to boil your own tap water and rehydrate with it.)

To cook at home, bring 1 cup of water to a boil with a pinch of salt, stir in ½ cup instant oats and simmer 3 minutes, then proceed as below.

	Ingredients	*Benefits*
1 bowl	cooked oatmeal	fibre; lowers cholesterol
1	banana, mashed	potassium powerhouse; reduces amt. of sugar
1 tbsp	white chia seeds	antioxidants/fibre/omega-3s
2 tbsp	hulled hemp seeds	pure protein, nutty flavour
2 tsp	pure maple syrup	better than "table syrup," which contains corn syrup and may spike insulin
½ cup	skim, 1% or 2% milk	calcium and comfort

Mash banana into oatmeal and stir in chia seeds and hemp hearts. Top with maple syrup and milk and feel awesome all day.

Preparation time: 3 minutes Serves: 2

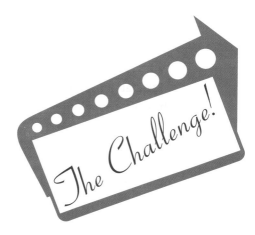

The Challenge!

YOU GET TO GO out for dinner! If that isn't in your budget right now, you can still do the challenge by deciding which restaurant you will go to when you are able or for a special occasion; pop in and ask for a menu or go online and make your imaginary decisions. Copy or tear out the Resto Rules pages and take them with you. This challenge is more fun with a pal, so bring someone who is willing to support you and learn too.

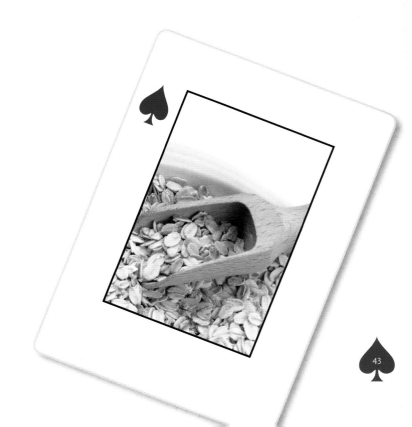

NINE OF SPADES

It can take no more than 20 minutes to get an entire week's worth of shopping done, honest! There is no guarantee that you won't be hung up in the cashier's aisle, but if you keep your regular shopping down to an automatic system, it can truly be a simple game. But, as with any game, there are rules.

Unless perusing the aisles for new products and reading labels is your thing, you need a routine to shop effectively. These tips will be explained in more detail in later chapters. For now, know that if you follow them, you are set up for success.

You have to know your brands in advance, who can you trust, and who's hoodwinking you. Being an avid label reader is a good thing but it adds to your time. As with any sports competition (and there's no question grocery shopping is a sport!), the best competitor prepares *before* the competition. Shaving your time means being trained and prepped and ready for the starting gun. As a general rule, you can't believe marketing claims like "fat-free" and "no trans fats." (The Five of Spades sheds more light on labels.)

Use this shopping session to buy your weekly food staples. This list guides you through the nine food aisles to get you through the week efficiently and healthily. Other items like packaged foods for lunches, laundry items, and paper products can be planned monthly.

Choose the same store over and over again, and don't be afraid to complain loudly each time they "reorganize to serve you better." This store should be a small, local grocer. You may save a few bucks at a big box store but the sheer size is intended to make you spend more — more time and more money. These mega-stores can be fun but if shaving time while staying healthy is your goal, save them for a rainy day and stock up then on everything you need.

Eat *before* you shop!

Make your decisions before the sliding doors greet you with blasts of temperature-regulated air and gentle music, lulling you into a slower pace. The music, by the way, is chosen specifically for certain times of the day. The stores know that moms shop during school hours and single gals and guys after 7 p.m. They play the music most likely to put you in a good (spending) mood.

Eyeball your progress by dividing the grocery cart into sections. The majority of the cart should be filled with items from the first five groups on the following list, primarily in the produce section. If you get this right at the grocery store, you can't help but fill half of your plate with fresh products.

The list below is ordered from most important to least. If you want more information, skip ahead to the playing cards noted.

PRODUCE (see Three of Spades). This is the only place where you will make decisions based on what's on sale, in season and looks good. Half of your time will be spent here. But don't mull for more than a minute; decide and move on.

Pick five green foods (for example, broccoli, spinach, kale, green onions, zucchini), four red/orange foods (peppers, squash, sweet potatoes), three blue/purple foods (blueberries, plums, red cabbage), two foods in the yellow spectrum (bananas, melons, green apples), one white food (onions or garlic).

FISH (see Jack of Hearts). You need to eat three servings of fish per week. Pick one fresh, in season or

on-sale species and some frozen shrimp or scallops. The third serving will come from canned tuna or salmon for lunch.

GRAINS (see Ten of Clubs). Brown rice (whole-grain quick-cook rice is fine) and quinoa.

ANIMAL PRODUCTS

- *Dairy* - Organic milk (see Nine of Hearts), butter (see Eight of Hearts), low-fat feta, low-fat mozzarella (grated), eggs, boxed egg whites.
- *Meat* (see Ten of Hearts) - choose one red meat meal per week. Make it lamb over beef as often as possible. Go for organic or grass-fed if affordable and/or available.
- *Chicken* (see Five of Clubs) - choose two or three cuts to use throughout the week.

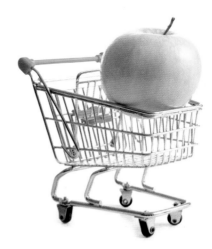

FROZEN FOODS. Whole-wheat tortellini, frozen shrimp or scallops, thin-crust pizza (whole-grain if possible), peas (green veg that most people like), Brussels sprouts (much more nutritious than peas), any other vegetables you like, 100 percent fruit juice concentrates.

BOXES, BOTTLES, AND CANS (see Seven, Six and Five of Spades). Crushed tomatoes, tomato paste, two types of canned beans plus a can of refried beans (because you are trying to have at least three meatless meals per week), curry sauce, quick-cooking oats and/or unsweetened oatmeal packets, whole-grain low-sugar breakfast cereal, canned skipjack tuna and/or salmon, canned sardines (see Jack of Hearts).

OILS (see Eight of Hearts). Extra virgin olive oil and grapeseed oil.

SPREADS (see Six of Spades). All-natural peanut butter, almond butter, hummus (sometimes in the produce section).

BAKED GOODS Whole-grain wraps, yeast-free bread, trans-fat-free oatmeal cookies. That's it. That is all it will take to get the average household through one week of breakfasts, lunches, and suppers that are healthy, simple, and delicious.

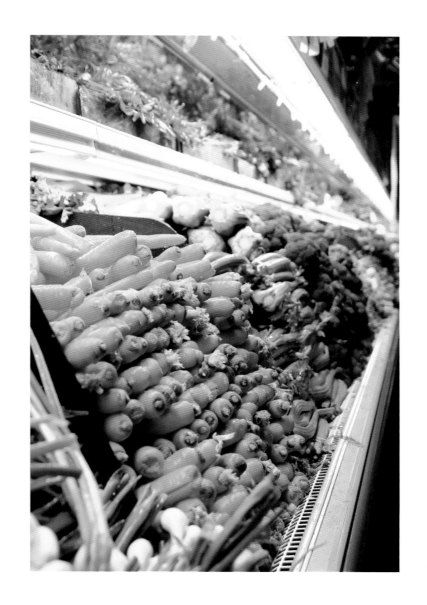

TRUMPED-UP 'ZA

In the time it takes to preheat the oven you can take a nutritionally ho-hum convenience food and turn it into a tasty, outstanding powerhouse of fuel. Most of the premade frozen pizzas have some toppings on them but the addition of a few truly nutritious ones makes for a more nourishing and substantial meal. This way, you can have one or two nutrient-dense slices, along with a salad, and feel satisfied, instead of filling up on the more calorie-dense, straight-out-of-the-box version. If you can't find a whole-wheat-crust pizza use a regular one.

Ingredients / *Benefits*

	Ingredients	Benefits
1	whole-grain frozen pizza	base for added healthy ingredients
1–3 tbsp	tomato paste	lycopene for prostate/heart health
1 tbsp	white chia seeds	antioxidants/fibre
1 tbsp	Italian seasoning	phytonutrients
1 cup	grated low-fat mozzarella cheese	calcium
	freshly grated black pepper	improves digestion; antibacterial
1 cup	baby spinach or arugula	lutein for vision

Preheat oven as directed on pizza package. Spread 1–3 tbsp of tomato paste onto frozen pizza and top with chia seeds, Italian herbs, mozzarella and black pepper. Bake for half the baking time required, top with spinach, bake the rest of the time.

Preparation time: 5 minutes Servings: 4

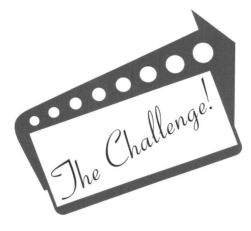

YOUR CHALLENGE THIS WEEK is to compare brands. You can do this in the store or online, wherever you are most comfortable and think you will get the most done. Choose two boxed products but make one a "healthier" brand and the other an economy brand. It's best to choose items from the granola bar, cookie, and frozen meals categories because they have wide variations in ingredients. You get bonus points for taking a minute to extrapolate information over a year. A brand of cookies with two more grams of fibre per serving may not seem like a lot but getting to your fibre goal of 25 grams per day may mean the difference between colon cancer, diverticulitis, or polyps. And choosing something like a high-fat lasagna (that has an extra 100 calories) daily may mean gaining an extra pound in a mere month. Do that for 12 months and what do you get?

ITEM	BRAND	CALORIES/ SERVING	SERVING SIZE	FIBRE	SODIUM
COOKIES					
LASAGNA					
PIZZA					

To really see the impact of this change, compare the numbers multiplied over a year's worth of consumption.

EIGHT OF SPADES

THE FREEZER SECTION: Must-haves for your freezer

One of the toughest parts about getting the eating thing right is the forethought that has to go into it. Many people go in to the grocery store without a plan and stumble out with various packages from the freezer section, referred to in the biz as "home-meal replacements" (HMRs). The name can be misleading because you might do better at home if you had the time. The lasagnas and the pizzas, as well as the more exotic pad thai and Indian offerings, are intended to save you time – all you need to do is pop them into the oven and walk away for an hour. I am encouraged by the number of frozen foods that continue to improve so if you read carefully and shop wisely the convenience can be yours.

Think about the "comfort foods" we have become accustomed to. The reason that they are comforting is that they require little or no effort to consume. The soft, warm *chew, chew, swallow* is what has gotten us into this mess in the first place. When you have to chew more, your brain perceives it is getting more food and registers satiety or fullness. The ease of soft, non-chew foods just makes us want to eat more.

Each mouthful ought to take you 10 to 15 chews to reach a swallowable size. That is a 200 or more percent increase in the energy spent just chewing the food! It really ought to take us 20 minutes or so to enjoy a plate of food. But most of our food is so soft (i.e., processed) that you can consume it mindlessly. And never is this more true than in the freezer aisle. I challenge you to find anything — low-fat healthy or highest-fat lasagna — that requires any chewing effort! Even if you can find the perfect HMR with low sodium, reasonable carbs and fats, I bet it wouldn't require you to actually chew.

Processing removes all of the effort of shopping for ingredients, cooking those ingredients, *and* consuming those ingredients. Time saving, yes, but at what cost if your body doesn't even know you have consumed them?

Compare a frozen pad thai meal to a homemade stir fry using whole-grain brown rice, which is quite chewy. Atop that bed of rice is a stir fry of crispy, stringy celery, and crunchy onions and peppers. Pieces of protein need to be pulled apart with the front teeth and then chewed at the back. You do have to work it a bit, right? Now, imagine topping that with a few peanuts or almonds. Nuts are one thing that people are careful to chew, and with good reason. We don't introduce nuts to toddlers for fear they will choke before they learn to fully masticate them. It will take you twice as long to eat this meal, and so it should.

I know, it will also take you twice as long to cook this meal and you don't have the time! No one is saying that we can't make the most of the convenience that is up for grabs in the freezer section. There are loads of time-saving secrets in there if you learn to shop smartly. Here is a list of nine foods that you do want from the freezer section. They are mostly single-ingredient foods that will add time to your day in a low-calorie way.

FOOD	HOW TO USE
Frozen shrimp or other cooked fish	Cooks in minutes, great for stir fries. Cook ½ cup whole-wheat pasta per person. Drain. In a skillet sauté for 4 minutes: ½ cup scallops/shrimp per person, 1 cup frozen peas per person, 1 tsp extra virgin olive oil per person, 1 tbsp Parmesan cheese. Add the cooked pasta and mix.
Frozen Brussels sprouts	Steam and toss with dill.
Frozen broccoli	Simmer 2 cups of broccoli and 1 potato in 1 quart of broth. Purée to soup consistency. Stir in 1 tbsp Parmesan cheese.
Frozen soybeans/lima beans	Steam for 2 minutes. Add seasoned rice vinegar. Makes a high-protein snack.
Frozen apple or pineapple juice concentrate	Replaces some sugar in baked goods with real fruit sugar (see recipe below for Pantry/Freezer Apple Spice Muffins).
Frozen whole-wheat tortellini	Great as a small portion loaded up with veggies (crushed tomatoes, sliced pepper and onions, etc.
Frozen berries	Irreplaceable superfoods in smoothies/baking.
Frozen pizza	Thin-crust and whole-wheat: add seeds, veggies, etc. (see Nine of Spades).

PANTRY/FREEZER
APPLE SPICE MUFFINS

Here is a muffin recipe that is simple and healthy. Not only does it use staple
ingredients that are probably in your pantry, it uses only whole–wheat flour,
is sweetened with applesauce and frozen 100 percent fruit juice, and contains only the good
fat from eggs. This is comfort food you can feel good about.

Ingredients

Amount	Ingredient	Benefits
2 ½ cups	whole-wheat flour	high-fibre; more nutrients than white flour
2 tsp	baking powder	makes muffins fluffy without adding fat
2 tsp	baking soda	eliminates need for added salt
2 tsp	allspice	aids digestion
½ tsp	nutmeg	cleans the liver, lowers blood pressure
2 tsp	cinnamon	regulates blood pressure/blood sugar
1	large pear or apple	pectin fibre; lowers cholesterol
12-oz can	unsweetened pineapple or apple juice concentrate	pure fruit sweetener
¾ cup	unsweetened applesauce	sugar-free vitamin C
1 tbsp	vanilla	traditional aphrodisiac
3	eggs	lutein and zeaxanthin; protect vision

Preheat oven to 375°F. Line a muffin tin with muffin papers. Combine all dry ingredients in a mixing
bowl and mix well. Grate pear or apple into bowl and toss to coat. Combine thawed pineapple
concentrate, unsweetened applesauce, vanilla, and eggs in a separate bowl. Pour into the dry
ingredients and quickly stir well. Fill tins to heaping and bake for 18–25 minutes. Muffins freeze well
for up to 6 weeks if tightly wrapped and are great for breakfast topped with almond butter.

Preparation time: 15 minutes Servings: 12

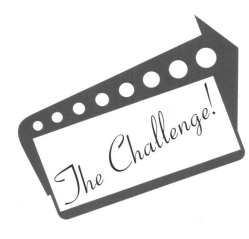

CREATE A RECIPE USING frozen shrimp or scallops. Per portion your recipe must have:

- at least one single-ingredient frozen food
- at least one cup of frozen shrimp or scallops
- at least two cups of vegetables (fresh or frozen)
- no more than one tablespoon of oil (grapeseed or sesame)
- no more than a half-cup of whole grains or whole food starch (rice, pasta or potato)
- no more than 300 milligrams of sodium (hint: soy sauce has almost 400 mg per teaspoon! You may want to look for an alternative product called Bragg's Liquid Amino Acids).

Recipe by: _____

Title: _____

MEASUREMENT   INGREDIENT

_____

_____

_____

_____

_____

PREPARATION METHOD

_____

_____

_____

_____

_____

_____

SEVEN OF SPADES

Ah, the pantry. Either you are blessed with a honking huge double door to dinner or you are, like me, in an urban setting with little space to spare. Either way there are some indispensable items that should be in your pantry, be it big or small, at all times.

I have chosen seven of my must-haves below. Most are nutrient-dense, delicious, affordable items that will stretch a meal in volume, nutrition, and taste.

CANNED TOMATOES

You will find the tomato sauce aisle shelved with the pasta and you should avoid it. Just look away. These jars seem to be the fastest route to a meal but there is a better, stronger, faster one to follow. The reason you want to walk away is that most canned pasta sauces and tomato sauces are so sodium loaded that you may be doing yourself more harm than good by eating them. Take a look at the label and if there are more than 300 milligrams of sodium per serving (most are more than 600 milligrams!), step away from the shelf. (If you can find one lower in sodium, I want to hear about it.) By contrast, in the canned vegetable aisle you can find canned tomatoes straight up, often unsalted. When you choose them, you are going a long way toward protecting your blood pressure, and avoiding belt buckle bloat. Tomatoes are high in vitamin A, iron, fibre, and the well-known nutrient lycopene and should be eaten two or three times per week. They are canned sunshine. If you choose the unsalted versions there are only five milligrams of sodium per half-cup. Even salt-added canned tomatoes have only around 300 milligrams per half-cup portion, which is a reasonable amount for a dinner meal. (You should consume only 2,000 to 2,500 milligrams per day; see Seven of Hearts.) It takes mere seconds to make your own tomato sauce for pasta dishes that tastes fresher, is better for you, and uses only the same pot you were going to use anyway (see recipe below).

TOMATO PASTE

This little dream can is a sodium-free and versatile antioxidant delivery system. If you can find tomato paste in a tube instead of a can, it is more convenient because you can use one teaspoon at a time and the rest can be refrigerated. Tomato paste should be added to every soup, sauce, and stir fry that you make. A little goes a long way in adding not only nutrients but colour and flavour. (And you learned in the Nine of Spades what it can do for frozen pizza.) (Salsa is great too, but we don't want to use up the whole list with tomato products, do we?)

CANNED TUNA AND SALMON

"But it's full of mercury!" Hear this: the benefits of eating fish still far, far outweigh the negatives of some mercury in your blood. Is mercury a problem? Yes! But there are ways to mitigate that risk. Plus, it turns out that selenium (a potent antioxidant being studied for its cancer-fighting properties) helps remove mercury from the body. Tuna and other fish are high in selenium. As well, there is news now that flaked or light tuna are from smaller fish that may not have accumulated much mercury. Mercury aside, fish is a lean protein that has good fats and good flavour and is cheap and quick. One can of tuna per week is fine. In the Jack of Hearts you will learn how to vary your fish sources and to eat as low on the food chain as possible to avoid mercury and other toxins. We should be lobbying for some ocean-protecting group to get our world cleaned up and stop blaming the humble fish.

MARINATED ARTICHOKE HEARTS

You probably don't know that artichokes are high in the important nutrients vitamin K and folate, as well as fibre. Plus, they are low in calories and are mildly anti-inflammatory. We used to say pickles are a dieter's best friend because they pack a flavour punch with relatively low calories but, boy, do they smack of sodium, and the bloating that ensues keeps the pounds packed on. Not so for artichokes. You can find them in jars, in a marinade that is mostly water and spices with a little bit of oil. They have fewer calories than olives and dress up any Mediterranean-type meal. Toss them into pasta sauce, onto pizzas, into salads, or just enjoy them on their own as a snack with your Friday night martini (see Four of Hearts).

PASTA

Here we go again with "What? I thought all carbs were bad for you." We need carbs and avoiding them means that your body will eventually rebel. The trick is to vary the type of pasta and the volume of what goes with it. For instance, your bowl should be two-thirds full of veggies and veggie-based sauce, and one-third full of pasta. Most of us do this the other way around. Plus, you can vary the types of pasta and not eat the white-wheat variety all the time. There are some whole-wheat pastas, but I have found that many people (especially kids) balk at the texture. The trick is to cook just one minute longer than the package instructs, which will soften the fibre so you hardly notice the difference. Try other types of pasta, too, such as kamut, brown rice, and quinoa. They are a little more expensive but you can use less of them and the higher protein content means that you don't have to add meat to get a balanced meal. In other words, better grain costs less than cheaper meat.

SAUERKRAUT AND ITS KOREAN COUSIN, KIMCHI

Many cultures have traditional foods that are fermented and fermentation turns out to have huge health benefits beyond just preserving an otherwise tasty, raw food, in this case, cabbage.

We all know that cabbage is good for us because it's high in fibre and vitamin A. We know that the antioxidants in strong-smelling cruciferous veggies (broccoli, cauliflower, Brussels sprouts, etc.) act as little cleaning crews. They run around your body sweeping out some of the naturally occurring DNA damage. You should try to eat fermented foods daily.

When you ferment cabbage you create the good bacteria that the gut uses to keep your system in balance and your immunity high.

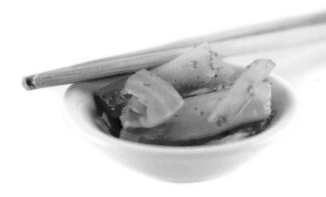

Similar to yogurt, fermented foods are crucial in keeping the bad bacteria down and the good ones up. The website *www.sauerkrautrecipes.com* has great ideas on how to use sauerkraut. The recipes range from soups using small amounts of cheap cuts of meat plus tomatoes and sauerkraut, through to Bloody Mary mixes and stuffed peppers. One of the easiest ways to work this food in is in sandwiches. Try filling a whole-wheat pita with one-quarter cup of grated jalapeno havarti and a half-cup of sauerkraut. Warm in the microwave for a minute and nosh. Kimchi is a little harder to find, but it is usually refrigerated with the Chinese noodles in the produce section.

CANNED PURE PUMPKIN

You *can* have dessert! Modify any pumpkin pie recipe (often right on the can), reducing the sugar by half. Bake the pie without a crust and serve it like a pudding. Or keep the crust, as long as it has no trans fats (hydrogenated vegetable oil or shortening) and eat only half of the crust half of the time.

Another creative way to use pumpkin is to stir a cup or two into spaghetti sauce. You won't taste it and it will thicken in a pleasing, high-nutrient way. Or you can serve it as a side dish. Pumpkin is no different from squash; simply warm it up, stir in a bit of butter and honey and maybe some salt and pepper. Serve in place of mashed potatoes.

ONE-POT TOMATO SAUCE

Almost as simple as opening a bottle of the premade stuff but way tastier and lower in sodium. If you divide this batch up into containers and freeze the leftovers, it will go a long way. For a smooth rather than chunky sauce, use puréed tomatoes instead of chopped and omit the tomato paste.

Ingredients

		Benefits
1 tbsp	grapeseed oil	boosts artery health
1	chopped onion, or 1 tsp dried minced onion	helps control blood sugar
2	cloves garlic, minced, or 1 tsp garlic powder	helps boost immunity
28-oz can	unsalted chopped tomatoes, drained	antioxidant
1 tsp	dried oregano	antibacterial
1tsp	dried basil	antibacterial
5.5-oz can	tomato paste	protects heart health
½–1cup	marinated artichoke hearts, drained	anti-inflammatory
	salt and freshly ground pepper, to taste	

In a large skillet over medium-high heat, warm oil (see Eight of Hearts). Add onion and sauté until translucent (about 5 minutes); stir in garlic. Add tomatoes to the skillet, with oregano and basil. Stir well. Simmer, uncovered, over low heat for 5–15 minutes. Stir in tomato paste and artichokes and warm through. Stir occasionally to prevent sticking. Season to taste with salt and pepper. Serve over kamut or whole-wheat pasta with a tablespoon or so of Parmesan cheese, if desired. Or better yet, use flaked yeast (see King of Spades).

Preparation time: 5 minutes Servings: 10

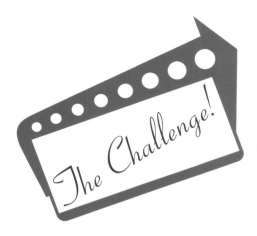
The Challenge!

CLEAN OUT YOUR PANTRY or cupboard. Take 20 minutes this week to remove all old cans or cans that contain less than stellar foods. Browse the labels for sodium content and get ready to be shocked! Anything (soups, canned pastas, sauces, etc.) that has more than 400 milligrams of sodium per serving is suspect and should be consumed with caution in small amounts. You really want to make some space for the single ingredient, truly good-for-you foods you will be eating from now on anyway.

SIX OF SPADES

BEANS: Toot sweet

The skinny on beans is twofold: they are a lean, low-cal, high-fibre protein in and of themselves, and the more often they are enjoyed in place of an animal protein, the more your calorie, fat, and cholesterol intake gets knocked down. When you replace a meal of animal protein with one of plant protein, you are consuming fewer calories, no cholesterol, and usually less fat. Plus, the more we eat primary-source protein (that is, it came right out of the ground and onto your plate rather than being first fed to an animal), the better off both the planet and its people are.

When most people think of beans they think of chili and nothing else and, while chili's good, it isn't best. To improve your chili, reduce the meat to minimal and bulk up the beans. Or better yet, make a completely meat-free chili (you can add texturized vegetable protein or tofu) — and please do not load up with cheese to make up for the missing meat!

The biggest complaint about beans is that they cause gas, but the more your bowel gets used to digesting these toot machines, the less musical they become. Like any muscle, the bowel needs the exercise of moving these starches and fibres. And just because black bean soup is a killer for you doesn't mean that lentil soup will be. Our guts have varying amounts of enzymes needed to digest different kinds of beans. Cheat on your favourite beans once in a while — sneak around with other varieties and see if you find any difference. You should be aiming for at least three meatless meals per week and the protein in beans is indispensable in achieving that goal.

Beans may also be the answer to a healthy liver, and a healthy liver is imperative for a healthy life. The liver conducts over 500 functions, ranging from cholesterol management to detoxification of body waste and pollutants (like wine, and also environmental toxins). The liver is the body's most regenerative organ and it works overtime. Not only does it clean up after the processes of life, it cleans up after itself and disinfects the

RECEIPT
City of Surrey
City Hall Parkade

License Plate Number

BA627E

Expiration Date/Time

08:38 PM
NOV 24, 2015

Purchase Date/Time: 07:38pm Nov 24, 2015

Total Due: $1.50
Total Paid: $1.50
Ticket #: 00003955
S/N #: 520014230461
Setting: City Hall Parkade
Mach Name: P1 Library

Rate: $1.50 for 1 Hour
Payment Type: Cash

Thank You

PARKING RECEIPT PARKING RECEIPT PARKING RECEIPT PARKING RECEIPT

NON TRANSFERABLE
Manufactured by T2 Systems Canada Inc.
Burnaby, B.C. Canada

Ace-D 4 D's
King-D 6C's
Queen-D 3B's
Jack-C
10-A 1A,
9-C
8-C
7-B
6-C
5-D
4-B
3-C
2-C
Bonus-Wild-B = Hearts

TERMS AND CONDITIONS
We accept no responsibility for loss or damage to vehicle or contents.
We do not take custody of vehicle but only rent space.

NON TRANSFERABLE
Manufactured by T2 Systems Canada Inc.
Burnaby, B.C. Canada

TERMS AND CONDITIONS
We accept no responsibility for loss or damage to vehicle or contents.
We do not take custody of vehicle but only rent space.

NON TRANSFERABLE
Manufactured by T2 Systems Canada Inc.
Burnaby, B.C. Canada

TERMS AND CONDITIONS
We accept no responsibility for loss or damage to vehicle or contents.

doorknob as it leaves. To support the liver, you need to drink lots of water, and take in nutrients like molybdenum. This trace mineral helps your liver to detoxify sulphites found in foods like wine, lunch meats, and medications. Hummus, which is made with chickpeas, just might be a hangover cure – but that's another story.

If that's not enough to convince you to eat more beans, consider how cheaply you can get them. A bag of dried beans is mere pennies a plateful and they are simple to cook: just soak them for eight to ten hours in two changes of water. Drain and empty into a slow cooker filled with water or boil in a large pot for an hour or two (depending upon the bean) and drain.

Draining reduces the fart factor and mustn't be skipped. Or open a can for a few pennies more. It is still cheaper than even the cheapest of meats. There are salt-free brands, but you can rinse away a significant amount of salt if you run the beans under cold water in a colander. Cultures all over the world have lived on beans and brown rice for centuries, and simple, delicious recipes can be found in Ethiopian, Indian, Mediterranean and Mexican cuisines, to name a few. It is worth a romp through Google to find a few new ones. Serving beans as a side dish in place of just about any rice, grain, or potato is a high-quality, high-protein way to control blood sugar.

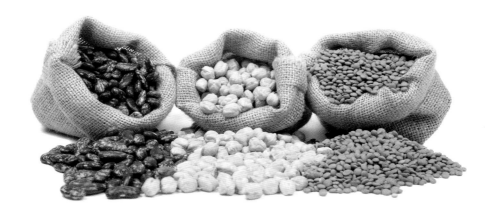

MEDITERRANEAN LENTILS

A great side dish in place of potatoes or rice. If you have a vegetarian in your house,
this dish supplies enough protein per serving to meet the daily requirement.
You could make this dish a few nights of the week without getting bored
if you kept changing the type of bean you use.

Ingredients

19-oz can	lentils
1 tbsp	extra virgin olive oil
2	garlic cloves, or 1 tsp powdered
¼ cup	grated Parmesan cheese
2 tbsp	nutritional yeast (optional)
	freshly ground pepper, to taste
	mixed herbs (thyme, basil, oregano, etc.),
	to taste

Benefits

fibre; lowers cholesterol

omega-9; lubricates arteries

vitamin B6; regenerates nerves

zinc; boosts immunity

probiotic; aids healthy digestion

boosts metabolism

trace minerals; support bone health

Drain lentils into a colander and rinse under cold water. Warm a cast iron skillet over medium
heat and add oil and garlic and quickly toss in drained lentils to keep oil temperature low. Stir for
1–2 minutes to heat through and mix in Parmesan cheese, nutritional yeast, and ground pepper.
Top with fresh or dried herbs to switch up the flavour.

Preparation time: 3 minutes Servings: 8

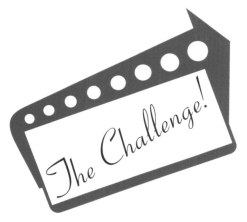
The Challenge!

BECOMING AWARE OF HOW much animal protein you eat is new for North Americans. It wasn't so long ago that dinner wasn't complete without a roast, lunch had meat sandwiches, and a really good breakfast had eggs and bacon. It was a source of pride to be able to afford to eat this way and we all thought that we needed this much daily protein. But we know better now. Plan ahead for three of your meals this week to be meat- (and egg-) free. Think about what you will use to replace that protein. (Hint: Other sources of protein are tofu, nuts, and beans.)

Bean burritos, for example, are easy as pie. Coat a tortilla with a smear of canned refried beans, add a handful of low-fat cheese, and warm in a pan. A tin of chickpeas tossed into a salad makes a great lunch.

	LUNCH	DINNER
MONDAY		
TUESDAY		
WEDNESDAY		
THURSDAY		
FRIDAY		
SATURDAY		
SUNDAY		

FIVE OF SPADES

READING LABELS: The secrets on, not in, the box

It's not surprising that we have become reliant upon snack food in packages – and who could blame us? With the speed of life cutting into our food prep time, who could possibly manage to have home-baked snacks and crackers week in and week out? So it is important to know exactly what is in that box and what to avoid. Is the truth really on the label?

Trust only the ingredient list, not the nutrition facts and not the health claims. This list has to be specific and it is ordered by ingredient from heaviest to lightest. Luckily, sugar and fat are heavy. Unluckily, there are many names for each, so "sugar" can be listed separately from "high fructose corn syrup." An important rule is that you must know what each ingredient is before you buy it. Real food looks and sounds like real food; it should be that simple.

The "Nutrition Facts" panel is flawed and complex. For instance, Health Canada has identified only calories and 13 "important" nutrients, chosen by a panel of experts. Fats (saturated and trans), cholesterol, fibre, sodium, carbohydrates, sugars, protein, calcium, vitamin A, vitamin C, calcium, and iron are listed. The problem is that groundbreaking work in nutrition isn't static and much has

happened *since* these labels were standardized, and the labels are not required to contain info on, for instance, magnesium, vitamin D, or omega-3. All are crucial elements of a well-nourished body and nutrients you want to maximize. But how can you maximize them if you don't even know they are there? Plus, under this system, the "good fats" are elusive and require a complex deduction of total fat minus trans plus saturated to decipher – way too complicated. Never mind the standing in the cookie aisle with a calculator. Ain't gonna happen.

Nutrition panels list nutrients per serving but serving size is set by the manufacturer and what you are actually eating may be way more. You may know how many servings of a particular food Canada's Food Guide recommends, but there is no requirement for a manufacturer to line up the recommendation on the package with the recommended serving size on the food guide. (Canada's Food Guide has its shortcomings but it is a fair place to start. You can pick one up in your doctor's office or go to the Health Canada website.)

Three-quarters of a cup of hummus is one serving of protein according to Canada's Food Guide, but you need to find a hummus that has less than 300 calories in that amount (and who eats that much hummus at a time, anyway?) or it's too caloric. Two tablespoons of a high-fat hummus may be the equivalent of consuming three-quarters of a cup of a low-fat one.

Ignore all marketing. That includes any banner saying "free of trans fats," "no trans," "zero trans," or any other fat claim. A manufacturer is allowed to use this claim providing that a product contains less than .2 grams of trans fats per serving. And we already know that they can mess with the serving size to fly under the radar. There is absolutely no need to have trans fats in our food at all! They are truly nasty stuff with no nutritional value and can do a lot of damage to your arteries. Many countries have already banned them outright, and there are products with healthier fats that taste just as yummy.

It is better to read the ingredients than the nutrition panel: they lie less. How do you think the skin of an orange would list its contents? "Orange." Or a package of walnuts? "Walnuts." Once you

learn this trick of focusing on the essentials, you can apply it easily in many aspects your life.

The goal of *Ace Your Health* is to help you balance real life by making lots of small shifts in your eating habits and outlook. Here are five guiding principles:

DON'T buy a snack food (cracker, cookie, granola bar, corn or potato chip) if:
- it contains more than 25 percent DV (daily value) of fat
- any trans fats are listed (except naturally occurring, as in milk)
- there are more than 200 milligrams of sodium per serving (and watch that you stay within that serving).

DO buy if:
- the fibre count impresses you with its heft; anything more than two to three grams is decent but you can get up to 12 to 15 in some. You need to get at least to 25 grams per day (see Queen of Clubs).
- the package has an expanded nutrition panel saying how much vitamin D, magnesium, or omega-3 it contains, as this non-mandatory nutrient information usually indicates things that are good for you.

HOMEMADE CRACKERS

This is a flexible, use-what-you've-got kind of recipe. And it's simple, so try it with your kids.

Ingredients — *Benefits*

1 cup	whole-wheat flour	manganese; for metabolism
¼ cup	amaranth (or rye or soy) flour*	added protein; regenerates cells
¼ tsp	baking powder	lends crispiness
¼ tsp	salt	cell balance
1 tsp	poultry seasoning	antioxidants
1 tsp	chili powder	boosts immune system
2 tbsp	butter	good fat for healthy hair
1 tbsp	olive oil	good fat for healthy skin
8 tbsp	water	helps kidneys process protein

(*optional, you can use 1¼ cups of whole-wheat flour instead)

TOPPING:

1 tsp	garlic powder	antibacterial
1 tsp	white pepper (or black)	enhances digestion
¼ tsp	herb seasoning mix	trace minerals

Preheat oven to 375°F. In a large bowl or food processor, mix together flours, baking powder, salt, poultry seasoning, and chili powder. Using your fingers or pulsing the processor, blend in butter and oil until the mixture looks like pellets. Drop water into dough by spoonfuls until the dough comes together and can be rolled out. Slice with a knife into 18–24 strips and lay on a baking sheet lined with parchment paper. Poke with a fork and sprinkle with garlic powder, pepper, and herb seasoning mix. Bake on top shelf for about 18–20 minutes. Store in airtight container for up to 10 days.

Preparation time: 25 minutes Servings: 10 to 12

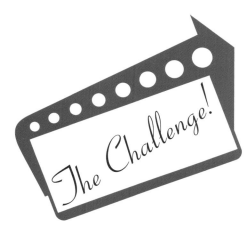

The Challenge!

GO TO YOUR SECRET snack cupboard (where you hide your personal Halloween stash) and find a package of your guiltiest pleasure. Or go to a grocery store or a friend's house. (This is one reason my friends shiver when I come over. They worry that if I find their secret stash I'll want to "help" them clean up their act.)

LOOK AT THE LABEL. Is there a marketing banner? What does it say? Now look at the ingredient list. Does it add up? If the word *hydrogenated* appears, there are trans fats in there, but in amounts small enough that the manufacturer doesn't need to disclose it on the panel.

COUNT HOW MANY WORDS end in *-ose* (glucose, fructose, etc.). These are all sugars that have been divided up by type so that they don't have to be listed as the first or second ingredient. Look at how many polysyllabic words there are. Do you know what any of those words mean? Chances are that they are fats or preservatives. In the case of some protein bars or cereals, there are added vitamins, but why do they need to be added anyway? Real food naturally contains vitamins.

LOOK AT THE SERVING size, measure out exactly that amount and decide if that is what you normally consume. Consume one serving. Throw the rest away and look for a better brand next time.

FOUR OF SPADES

CONTAGIOUS BEHAVIOUR:
How you really do get by with a little help from your friends

———————

"Show me your friends and I will tell you who you are" was a phrase my father uttered frequently that infuriated me as a fiercely independent teen. "I am an individual who makes her own choices," I would tell him. "My friends don't influence me. I can think for myself. *Sheesh!*"

But I can now see that it's true, and there is proof. A doctor and a behavioural scientist studied "social contagion" using data from the Framingham Heart Study, the longest-running study of heart disease so far. Framingham started in 1948 (and is still ongoing, with its third cohort of descendants) and tracked 15,000 people in a town in Massachusetts. It has been a wealth of information far beyond its original intended purpose of understanding the influences and onsets of disease.

The researchers used the Framingham data to draw connections between people. They found that people grew fatter (or not) in clusters depending upon with whom, within the study, they were connected. We wouldn't have needed a study to tell us that if we'd listened to our fathers. And we've all seen average-weight children with overweight parents pack on pounds. It makes sense: they are in the same household, eating the same stuff and getting the same amount of exercise — and they started with the same genes. But it *is* a revelation that those heavy parents probably hang with other heavy people. According to this study, we socialize according to our commonalities. So, even though tennis-playing Susan lives next door to chip-eating Lucy, they aren't likely to be friends. Susan doesn't want to eat chips and watch movies all the time, and Lucy doesn't want to swing a racquet at the tennis club.

The data suggest other, less obvious connections. For instance, it was discovered that we have three degrees of influence. That means our behaviour influence can skip a link. A shift in Susan's behaviour may not influence Lucy, but Lucy's daughter is watching from next door and she may be influenced.

The study also showed that smoking, drinking, happiness, and loneliness may have a social connection component. The theory is that there are subconscious social signals that we pick up from those around us that serve as cues for normal behaviour. It is a lot like the herd behaviour seen in schools of fish, herds of horses, flocks of geese, etc. No one really tells the herd, "We are going left"; there is no sound or memo, someone simply makes a subtle shift, which passes to the next and the next, until the whole group veers. Beautiful to watch, and replicable in our own lives.

It is troubling to see portrayals of overweight children in kids' media. Animated movies and advertisements that portray pudgy children are probably meant to be inclusive, but the result may be to *normalize* being overweight. Luckily, this influence cuts both ways. It is inspiring to know that your reading this book on the bus may pique someone's interest enough for them to make healthy changes. Telling two friends about this book may not change their behaviour, but they may hear about it again in another setting and think: "Hey, my friend loves that book!" which may make yet someone else get in on the game.

We need to choose our friends wisely and use our internal compass to guide them as they guide us. We need to gather with those who inspire us more often. We need to laugh away some stress, enjoy some social connection, and encourage good eating. The idea isn't to dump your fat friends but rather to teach them by example. It's the swapping of ideas and taking the time to follow through that matter significantly to our health. Life is just way more fun when you have a handful (or a herdful) of people who enjoy you as you enjoy them.

ROAST CHICKEN DIJON

No matter which theme you choose (unless it's vegetarian!) for a dinner party, this easy roast chicken will fit in. The flavours are bold enough to be tasty but simple enough to go with anything. Roasting a whole chicken saves time and money; it takes mere moments to get it into the oven and then you can walk away. If you have loads of friends, roast two, or three and count yourself lucky.

Ingredients

		Benefits
1	3–4 pound roasting chicken	selenium; fights cancer
1 cup	white wine	resveratrol; protects telomeres
3 tbsp	grainy Dijon mustard	selenium; anti-inflammatory
1 tsp	cracked black pepper	aids digestion
2 tbsp	apple cider vinegar	helps absorption of minerals
1 tbsp	thyme leaves	aids digestion
1 tsp	garlic powder	antimicrobial

Preheat oven to 375°F. Mix white wine, mustard, pepper, vinegar, thyme, and garlic together and pour onto and into the chicken. Place, breast side up, in rack in roasting pan. Bake chicken in oven for 2–2½ hours, or until internal temperature reaches 185°F. Allow to sit for 5 minutes before carving. Leftovers can be stored in the fridge up to 3 days and are great in salads for lunch.

Preparation time: 10 minutes Servings: 6

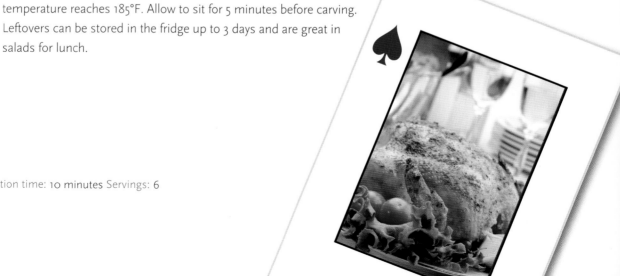

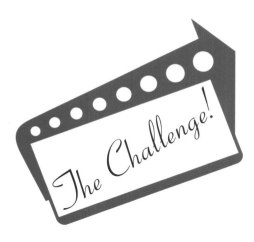

The Challenge!

GATHER THE GANG AND have a healthy potluck party. Make this an opportunity to engage some colleagues, book club members, or neighbours that you see in the hallway or driveway. Spread the good habits!

Pick a meal time: (brunch, dinner, breakfast, tea time . . .)

_____

Pick a theme: (red food, round food, holiday food, ethnic food . . .)

_____

Make a guest list:

FOOD CATEGORY	GUEST NAME	DISH
SOUP		
APPETIZER		
SALAD		
VEGETABLE		
VEGETABLE		
BEAN SIDE DISH		
DESSERT		
PROTEIN		

THREE OF SPADES

VEGGIES AND FRUIT: The anatomy of a salad

We all know that fruits and vegetables are good for us, that's not news. But science is only now revealing the deeper truth of that statement and what, exactly, is in each one that is such a benefit to us. We could focus on all the things you must eliminate from your life to be healthy, but I much prefer to focus on what you can *add*.

Where else in life is it really true that more is better? The good news is that vegetables are low in calories, high in water, and delicious just as they come out of the ground. You can't eat too much or too many. The one caveat is that fruit has more sugar and thus more calories and should be enjoyed in abundance without overdoing it.

Vegetables and fruit can be grouped by colour and coded by which antioxidants they contain and what they can do for you. Here's your crib sheet.

Red fruits and vegetables like tomatoes and strawberries contain *lycopene* and *anthocyanins* to protect your heart, memory, and urinary health.

White fruits and vegetables like onions, leeks, and garlic contain sulphides and *allicin* to protect your heart and keep your blood pressure in a healthy range.

Blue fruits and vegetables like blueberries and purple cabbage contain *phenolics* to protect your joints and brain.

Yellow or orange fruits and vegetables like oranges and squash contain *carotenoids* to boost your immunity and protect your vision.

Green fruits and vegetables like spinach contain *lutein* and *indoles* to protect your bones, teeth, and eyes.

They all contain fibre, minerals, and vitamins. In addition, they contain antioxidants, which are the tools the plant uses to protect itself from predators and drought. Learning how to deal with its environment forces the plant to armour itself. This armour becomes the antioxidant, antimicrobial, antifungal agents that do us so much good when we ingest them. They have protected the plant from its external environment which, in turn, helps us protect our internal environment. "What doesn't kill you makes you stronger" goes for vegetables and people. There is no scientific consensus over what is better for us, organically grown or conventionally grown food. The full and specific definition of organically grown depends upon the country of origin and the crop being discussed. For our purposes, let's define organic as "grown without the use of pesticides and herbicides and grown in soil rather than hydroponically (in water)." Everything else is conventional. Deciding on which way to go is a personal choice that depends upon your access to these foods, your finances, and your priorities. The issue isn't that conventionally raised foods contain pesticides – which can often be washed off – though that's part of it; it is that they can contain fewer phytonutrients (plant compounds that have beneficial health effects).

Think of it this way: the more nutrients that the soil can give to the plant, the more the plant has for you. In addition, the harder that the plant has to struggle to survive and grow, the stronger it will be and it can pass on that strength to you.

When figuring out the benefits of a fruit or veg, you have to consider two things: what kind of soil it was grown in and what kind of treatment it received to get it to market. The soil itself might be depleted in nutrients that the plant needs to make strong antioxidants and fertilizer may have been used to supply missing nutrients. A commercially and artificially fertilized plant may *look* almost the same but it may be different on the cellular level. Fungicides may have been used to combat mould, so the plant did not have to make the necessary phytochemicals. It is these chemicals that are helpful to our bodies.

Having fully armed, experienced plants in your salad bowl so you can build stronger cells to deal with life's illnesses and deficiencies is the goal. Of course, conventionally raised vegetables are good for you; the benefits of these still exist and in spades! For my money, I buy organic greens whenever I can and as much other organic produce as I can when it's on sale or close in price. The dark leafy greens are the power-packed workhorses of the vegetable family, and if I could have only one organic green it would be spinach. It cooks quickly, works as a salad, and is affordable and available.

Eat as many vegetables of as many colours as humanly possible each and every day. Aim for one huge salad at lunch every day this week. If you have to pack it, you may need two or three containers to hold the amount of salad I mean by "huge."

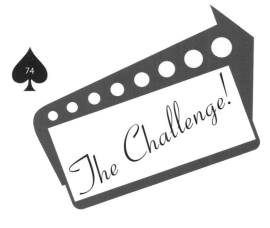

The Challenge!

THIS WEEK THE CHALLENGE and the recipe are the same: to eat one salad daily, with each one containing all four colours. Assemble it from a salad bar or from your own fridge, but no days off! Keep track of what you put on your salad, choose from every category and see if you can get your score up to 100.

Points

1. Four handfuls of any mixture of (preferably organic) greens:
    raw spring mix, baby spinach, arugula, romaine, dandelion,
    cabbage, steamed asparagus, broccoli, or kale   **20**

2. Any mixture of ½ cup of red or white vegetables:
    roasted red peppers, pickled beets, pickled hot peppers,
    chopped pickled vegetables, radicchio, radishes   **10**

3. Any mixture of blue fruit:
    blueberries, plums, figs, grapes, blackberries,
    black currants   **10**

4. Four to five ounces of any protein:
    1 cup canned chickpeas (or other beans, rinsed),
    1 tin canned tuna,1 tin canned salmon, some
    leftover chopped meat (1 chopped chicken breast,
    sliced of steak, chopped fish), 2 tbsp hemp seeds,
    1 boiled egg   **10**

5. Good Fats (pick one or mix and match portions of each!):
    ¼ avocado, 1 tbsp extra virgin olive oil, 1 tsp hemp seed oil,
    2 tbsp nuts, 1 tbsp grated cheese   **5**

6. Bonuses:

Squeeze of fresh lemon or lime	3
White chia	10
Fresh herbs	2
Black pepper	2
Dried herbs	3

7. Subtract 10 points for every item below: **-10**

Mayonnaise or bottled dressings

Tuna or salmon or egg "salad" (i.e., mixed with mayo)

Cheese as a "protein"

Croutons

Corn chips

Tortilla "bowl"

Chow mein noodles

Unmeasured amounts of fat

Cheeseburger and fries (ha!)

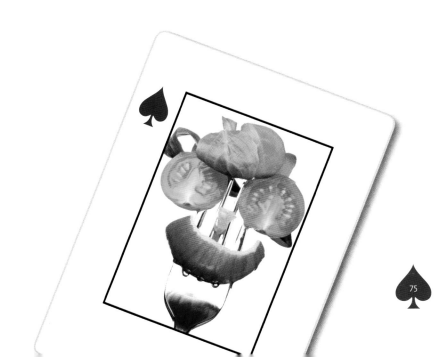

75

TWO OF SPADES

FAST FOOD: Drive through, please

_____

Okay, I do it too. I drive through . . . wearing a ball cap and dark glasses and disguising my voice. So let's look at the ways to cope when life throws us into a day that can't be managed without a stranger handing us a brown paper bag through a window.

There are loads of options for on-the-road dining, we just don't think of them. For instance, it is just as fast (and a bit healthier and cheaper) to pull into a grocery store, grab a packaged salad and some grilled chicken strips. But on a road trip, sometimes the easiest way to refuel is at one of the top five fast-food restaurants: McDonald's, Tim Hortons, Wendy's, Burger King, and Harvey's. (Subway can be a good choice too but most do not have drive-throughs.) I am not a huge fan of any of them, but they do fill the gap and, with a little help, you can make better choices. They've all made improvements in the last decade and now post nutritional info on their websites. McDonald's is even working toward having their info on their packaging. Having the information to make good decisions is what *Ace Your Health* is all about.

Here is the scenario. You are on the road and take an exit off the highway where all five of these drive-through choices await you. Which do you choose? This assessment looks at which items on each menu net the most nutrients and health-promoting phytonutrients per calorie with the lowest sodium count. The goal is to keep the belly full as healthily as possible until you can get a real meal. This stop-gap way of eating should be used as sparingly as possible — no more than once per week. And following my Number One Rule (nothing deep-fried) means no French fries. Sorry.

There were no choices available, even on the best of the menus, that did not serve up half a day's worth of sodium in just one meal. A well-nourished body needs three meals and two snacks in a day, and if you eat frequently at fast-food places, there's no way to keep your sodium intake within healthy limits (1,000 to 2,000 milligrams a day).

TIM HORTONS

A Canadian institution, and who doesn't love their coffee? But choosing Tim's means foregoing the fat- and sugar-laden doughnuts. Unfortunately, for lunch or dinner choices, Tim's takes the salt cake. Have no part of their soups or chili – the salt content would shock you (e.g., 1,320 milligrams in the chili). Instead, have a Barbecued Chicken Wrap (whole-wheat, a road rarity!), ask for extra lettuce and tomato and grab a steeped tea, black (see Queen of Spades) and a low-fat yogurt and berries. You'll be back on the road after 350 worthwhile calories and only about 30 percent of your daily intake of sodium. Of all the drive-through options, this is your best bet.

MCDONALD'S

Grilled Chicken Snack Wrap, with grilled (not crispy!) chicken, and a side Garden Fresh Salad will net you under 400 calories and 35-50 percent of a day's worth of sodium. That includes just *half* a pack of Asian Sesame Dressing. If you really have to have a burger, order a Junior Burger and throw away half the bun.

WENDY'S

Baked Potato with Broccoli and Cheddar Cheese with a Junior Burger gets you the most nutrients for your approximately 600 calories and 50 percent of a day's worth of salt. Go topless: throw away half the bun and save 60 calories and 100 milligrams of sodium.

BURGER KING

You are going to have to trade off fat for sodium and choose either the Veggie Burger (for less fat and more sodium) or a hamburger (for more saturated fat but less sodium). Each is about 310 calories but if you throw away half the bun and load up on tomatoes, mustard, onions, and lettuce, you will hardly miss it. You can add a side salad, with a half-packet of any dressing you want (the light ones have too much salt and the creamy ones too much fat – pick your poison) and enjoy it as long as you avoid the croutons; finish with an applesauce and you'll have a pretty decent nutrient count for your 450 calories and almost 50 percent of daily sodium.

HARVEY'S

Your best bet here is the Veggie Burger provided you opt out of BBQ sauce or "light" mayo. Stick with ketchup, mustard, relish, extra lettuce, tomato, and onions, and you are doing okay on the calories at about 350 but at about half of the maximum intake of salt. A side salad should fill you up and the best dressing option is the Asian Sesame, but it weighs in at 60 calories and 264 milligrams of sodium. The less you use, the better.

BARBECUED CHICKEN WRAP

Be it road picnic or regular lunch box, cooked chicken is an easy, portable lean protein. You can have all the taste and ease of a takeout meal with none of the downside. Scale up the recipe to make extra for the entire week and you will have your own homemade fast food.

Ingredients

		Benefits
6 ounces	boneless, skinless chicken thighs (or breasts or firm tofu)	lean protein
1 tsp	grapeseed oil	less damaged by heat
¾ cup	frozen corn	high fibre
2 tbsp	barbecue sauce	tomato-based; adds flavour
½ cup	roasted red peppers, chopped	vitamin A for eyes
2	whole-wheat tortillas	fibre without yeast
6	romaine lettuce leaves, or 2 cups mixed greens	folic acid; promotes cell division
1 tbsp	grated part-skim-milk mozzarella cheese	low-fat source of calcium

Warm a skillet over medium heat while you chop the chicken or tofu. Add oil to skillet and cook chicken 5–8 minutes. Thaw corn in microwave, drain, then add to skillet. Add barbecue sauce and red peppers. Stir to mix. Place tortillas flat on counter and layer with lettuce, skillet mix and cheese. Roll tortilla. (If packing for later use, allow chicken to cool before wrapping.) Wraps store well in the fridge up to 3 days. For a healthy packed lunch, serve with an apple or pear and a Tetra Pak of 100 percent juice.

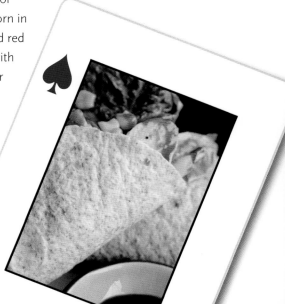

Preparation time: **15 minutes** Servings: **2**

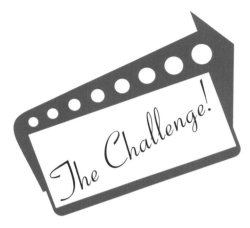

The Challenge!

PICK ONE OF YOUR favourite drive-throughs and tally up your usual meal using the nutritional charts posted online. Imagine disassembling the items and stuffing any veggies and fruit into measuring cups. How many cupfuls of truly nourishing phytonutrients from plant-based foods would you get? (You need at least two full cups at this meal to keep up with your daily requirement.) None for a burger and fries! Any dairy or other calcium, like almonds, broccoli, cheese? Not likely!

MENU ITEM	CALORIES	FAT (g)	SODIUM (mg)	FIBRE (g)
TOTAL MEAL				

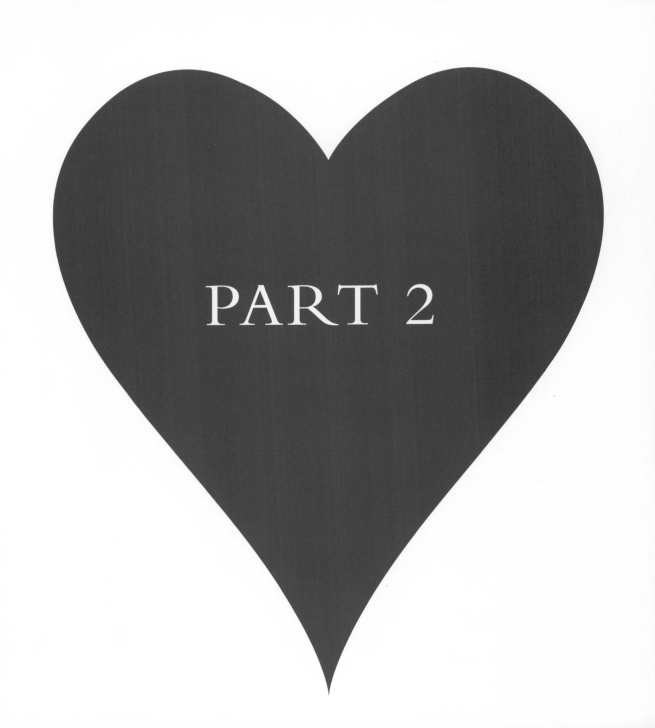

PART 2

*N*ow that you have a solid foundation of the key ways to build your health, wouldn't it be great to be alive to enjoy it? Nothing stops a life from being lived faster than a heart that stops beating. Heart disease is a huge issue, mostly because of our lifestyle choices around food, exercise, and stress. The good news is that many of these factors are within our control and can be changed: we can eat heart-healthy foods, we can be active, and we can manage our stress. So why don't we? Often the answer is that the speed of our everyday lives makes the task seem overwhelming. This section lays out simple, practical plans and challenges to strengthen your heart through good choices. One by one, you will make some big changes without feeling deprived or overwhelmed. By the end of 13 weeks, if you fulfill each challenge, you will be well on your way to a healthier heart. The Hearts section offers a positive proactive approach to keeping that ticker ticking – one that you can do even while you sleep.

ACE OF HEARTS

EXERCISE: At the crossroads

A recent study by the U.S. Institute of Medicine, an independent, non-profit organization that works outside of government to provide unbiased and authoritative advice to decision makers and the public, concluded that we need to have a minimum of 60 minutes of vigorous exercise every day to positively affect our cardiovascular health. Try not to perceive this guideline as a mountain too tall to scale and give up right now. Hear me out.

Humans are designed to move all day, every day, but in our modern world we don't. Our grandparents would have knocked off that one hour of exercise easily, just in the normal course of getting out of bed to milk the cows or walk to the factory. Fitting a trip to the gym into our busy days may feel completely unrealistic. But you don't have to start with such a big step. You will benefit from any additional movement you add to your day. If you are in your thirties, forties, or fifties with a family history or personal experience of heart disease, you need to get your keister off the couch!

Keep in mind that every load of laundry you carry up the stairs or 15 minutes that you walk the dog counts in burning off the calories you consume. Every yoga class and game you coach (and I mean on the ice, field, or court, not screaming from the stands!) is movement. When you accept that human beings are meant to move for eight to ten hours per day, the required one hour of exercise doesn't seem so impossible. Rather, it is the first and best step in protecting your heart.

But it isn't only the heart that benefits from exercise. Countless studies illustrate the positive effects of exercise on concentration, sense of well-being, cardiovascular health, and even cancer.

One recent study looked at how much exercise was necessary to *protect* our cancer-protecting cells (telomerase; see Ace of Clubs). In other words, is more better? Exercise is a stress reliever but it also stresses the body. When we exercise, we are working harder and our cells have to replace and repair themselves more quickly. Which is good, but the wear and tear takes its toll. Too much exercise means that the repair costs are too great. The conclusion in this study was that burning anywhere between 1,000 and 2,400 calories per week is the sweet spot. More than that is too stressful on the body.

If getting some, but not too much, aerobic exercise is our goal, the first step in our strategy is to gain knowledge.

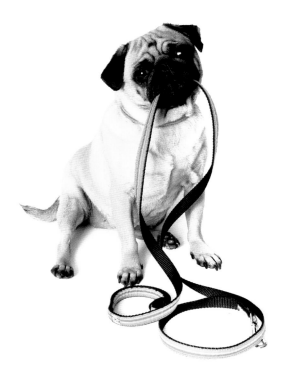

DARK CHOCOLATE SHAKE

As a reward before or after exercise, this dark chocolate shake is the perfect "rev me or replenish me" drink. Hemp protein powder can be found in the health food section of the grocery store, and it is a better choice than soy or whey because it has a more complete amino acid profile, plus GLA (gamma-linolenic acid) and chlorophyll (which is what makes it green, and why we hide it with cocoa!). If you can't find hemp protein powder, use unsweetened soy or whey powder.

Ingredients

		Benefits
2 cups	skim milk (or soy or rice milk)	vitamin D; builds bones
1	banana	potassium; electrolyte recovery
2 tbsp	pure maple syrup	mineralized carbohydrate; replaces glycogen in muscles
2 tbsp	hemp protein powder	repairs muscles
1 tbsp	cocoa powder	repairs telomeres
1 tsp	cinnamon	regulates blood pressure

Place all ingredients in a blender and blend until smooth.

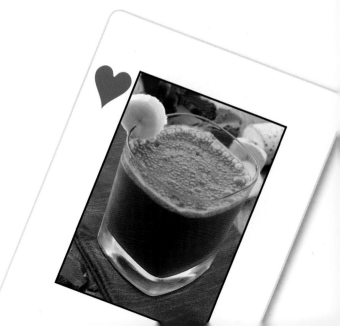

Preparation time: 2 minutes Servings: 2

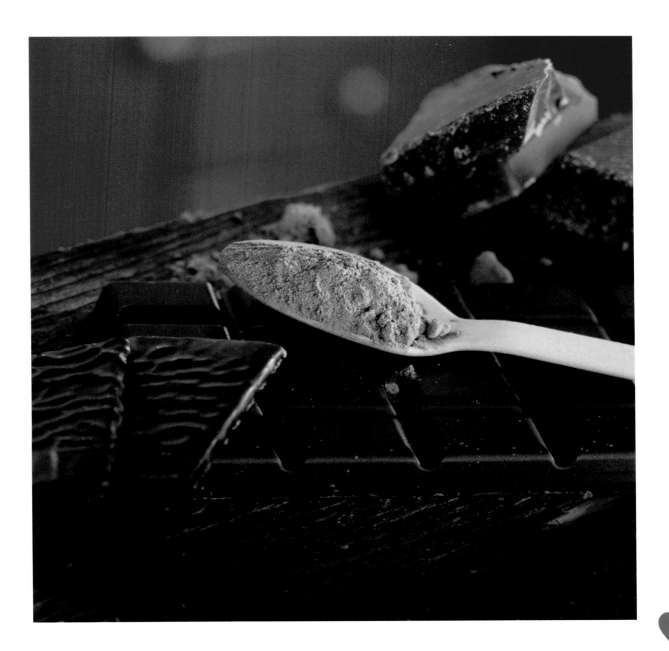

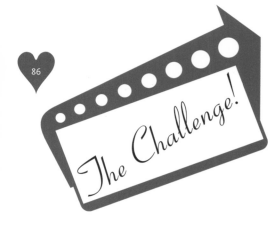

The Challenge!

REMEMBER AND RECORD THREE activities you liked to do when you were a teen. Running? Tennis? Hockey? Hiking? Rowing? If you didn't exercise as a teen, think of activities you might enjoy now.

1. _____

2. _____

3. _____

Make a decision to bring one of these activities back into your life. Don't turn the page just yet! Stay with me here. It's just a decision for now. Nothing else needs to happen . . . yet. Just write down: "I have decided to get more activity into my life by _____." By doing this you are agreeing that you need to expect a little more from yourself if you are going to live a life that is both happy **and** healthy.

Now take out your agenda or calendar. Schedule in everything that you will be doing over the next week, from the moment you open your eyes to the moment you crawl into bed. Include commute times and the time that you spend relaxing, such as watching TV, playing video games, social networking, or anything that you do sitting down while you are not working.

Circle all of the "relaxing items" or holes in your calendar. We have come to your crossroads. Take one hour of those "relaxing" things every day and replace it with an activity that you like to do. If your circled items are all in the evening and you are wiped out in the evening or don't like to go out in the dark, then you have some time shifting to do. There are 24 hours in every day and seven days in every week, 168 hours in total – you are only looking for seven!

Of course, it takes time to drive to the gym or lace up the skates or strip down to your tank top and basketball sneaks, but if you love it enough you will do it. And, if you remember your goal (a long life without illness or burdening your loved ones), you will make activity a priority. I have never heard anyone say they regretted exercise after they have done it. Think yourself through to that moment, not the current one of inertia. Once activity is in your schedule, protect it; don't rethink it each and every time.

You need to build from your starting point. If you already have at least an hour of exercise incorporated into your day, try to increase your workout time by five minutes a day each year or increase the weight you're lifting by 2 percent or your intensity by one level.

If you are just getting in the game, know that you are not alone. Build up to one hour slowly by starting with 10 minutes of stretching on the floor in front of the TV. Next week you will be limber enough to go for 15 minutes. Next month that stretching will turn into walking . . .

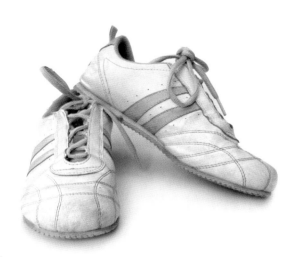

KING OF HEARTS

NON-EXERCISE ACTIVITY THERMOGENESIS: That's so NEAT!

Non-Exercise Activity Thermogenesis (NEAT) refers to every calorie you burn outside the gym or the playing field. Studies show how much our NEAT has changed in the last 50 years. As many kinds of activity have decreased, our pant sizes have increased.

Think of how much work it took to do the laundry when your mother or grandmother had to use a wringer washer! Hauling, lifting, stirring, feeding through the wringer, hanging on the line, and folding every piece of clothing took hours of toil. It was a pain in the pants, but that's the point! No matter what our mothers or grandmothers ate, they burned it off during the normal course of a day. Imagine what our grandfathers had to do to till the soil. Just hooking up the horses probably burned more energy than it takes you to get into the car, commute to the city, park underground, and stand in line for a coffee before getting to your desk.

Now think about all of the movements that we have cut out of our lives. We take the escalator instead of the stairs, we push the handicap button to open a door, and we use the remote control for pretty much everything from turning on a gas fireplace (not even the effort of building a wood fire!) to the TV and the ceiling fan.

A study done at the renowned Mayo Clinic took healthy volunteers and overfed them by 1,000 calories per day for eight weeks. The results showed that not all of them gained weight, and that some people unconsciously compensated to avoid doing so, for instance, by maintaining better posture or fidgeting. Even people who are demonstrative with their hands while talking burn more calories than those who are still, which makes simple sense. But we can't all become arm-waving, foot-tapping fidgeters overnight.

Here are a few things you can do that will make a difference in the long run:

For the entire time that you are getting ready in the morning, stand up tall. It is easy to slouch over the coffee maker, but if you knew that simply correcting your posture (more specifically, the minor effort that it takes to do so) could burn off calories, why wouldn't you? Put on your slippers, square your shoulders, and march to the loo, swinging your arms. No one can see you who hasn't see you do all sorts of weird things already. It will make you giggle, sure, giving you the right mindset for the day.

When you get to your desk, how do you sit? Is it possible to have a stability ball in your space? If so, spend the first hour of the day balancing on this ball instead of slumping over your computer with your chin on your wrist. (Oh, wait, that's me; my massage therapist explained that's what is probably causing the pain in my left shoulder blade.)

When you are ready for lunch at work, take the stairs down. C'mon, it's down, not even up! Walk around the building once, on your way to the lunchroom, whistling while swinging your arms and squaring those shoulders again. What else could you do that wouldn't cost you any time in your day?

- Take the stairs at the subway, just once a day, one flight.
- Shake your foot during a long meeting.
- Stand up for 20 minutes on a long phone call.
- Tap your pencil on your desk (as long as it doesn't drive anyone else crazy!).
- Flick your hair off your shoulders two extra times.
- Always push the door, don't use the handicap button.
- Use a basket at the grocery store instead of a cart.
- Squeeze your butt cheeks while sitting on the bus. No one's watching, they're all slumped in their seats, not using their NEAT to their advantage!

You would be surprised how these simple movements burn up body fat and build muscle and bone.

SUN-DRIED TOMATO EGG PUFFS

This is a delicious, low-cal, nutrient-dense recipe for breakfast, lunch, or snacks.
Whipping the eggs by hand will activate some NEAT; don't use an electric mixer.
One minute per arm and you – and the eggs – are good to go. Serve three puffs
per meal with salsa on the side and a glass of carrot juice or vegetable juice.

Ingredients		*Benefits*
1 carton	egg whites	lean protein
1 tbsp	sun-dried tomatoes, chopped	scavenges free radicals*
1 tbsp	white chia seeds	soluble fibre; lowers cholesterol
½ cup	plain yogurt	phosphorus; for pH balance
pinch	cayenne pepper	capsaicin; reduces inflammation
pinch	sea salt	mineral-rich and unprocessed
1 cup	salsa (on the side)	low-cal; high in vitamin C

Preheat oven to 425°F. In a large bowl, whisk egg whites for about 2 minutes.
Drain the sun-dried tomatoes and squeeze with paper towel to absorb most of the oil.
Chop and whisk tomatoes into eggs, along with chia seeds, yogurt,
cayenne, and salt. Use the oily paper towel to grease a 12-count
muffin tin. Divide the mixture among the muffin cups, taking care
to distribute tomatoes evenly. Bake for 8–12 minutes until puffed,
slightly browned, and cooked through.

And make a difference over a month or a lifetime.

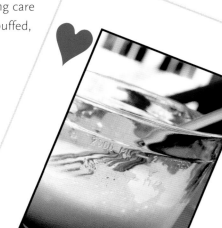

Preparation time: 9 minutes Servings: 4

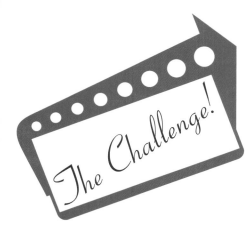

The Challenge!

THIS WEEK, TRY OUT five NEAT activities that don't cost time or money, but speed up your metabolism, even just a bit.

1. _____

2. _____

3. _____

4. _____

5. _____

QUEEN OF HEARTS

SLEEP: You are only as good as last night's Zzzzs

The jury is in: driving drowsy is as dangerous as (if not more so than) driving drunk. And yet millions of us do it every day. We bolster ourselves with caffeine and keep going – there's just so much to be done!

All together, as a population 21 percent of us use some kind of painkiller, tranquillizer, or sleeping or anti-anxiety pill. We're all hoping for a better night's sleep, and yet we soldier on with our bad habits.

Here are some of the common things that interfere with your sleep:

1 CAFFEINE: Caffeine gets a chapter all to itself; it is too big to bully into one paragraph (see Queen of Spades).

2 INDIGESTION: Eating too late at night interferes with your sleep. It isn't so much that you have heartburn or that "full feeling" keeps you awake, which are both true, but it is more about what your body is being asked to do. When you sleep, hormones are released. They have the "reboot" role and eating, especially a large heavy meal, interferes with their work of repairing cell damage.

3 STRESS: Stress is a huge factor in not getting a good sleep and you need to be aware of your state of mind right before you hit the hay. Sitting in front of a flickering computer or TV screen, balancing your chequebook, or fighting with the neighbour are not restful activities. There is a process that your body needs to go through before it lets itself relax. Think of it as sleep foreplay. A warm bath, journal writing, 20 deep breaths, and a quick peek at pictures of your vacation, rather than the corporation's spreadsheet, all do wonders.

4 VIGOROUS EXERCISE AT NIGHT: Don't get me wrong, exercise is great for you! But because it heats up your metabolism long after you stop exercising, it's hard for your body to switch gears into a restful state. That's when you might notice that you aren't sleeping well and turn to caffeine to stay awake through the day (which takes you back to the top of this list). It's a vicious cycle. Still, the benefits of exercise outweigh the negatives of doing it at night. So if the only time you can exercise is at night, try to finish at least three hours before you expect to sleep. Or try moving exercise to the morning on weekends. Then the benefits will last all day and all night.

⑤ LACK OF MAGNESIUM: It takes calcium to flex a muscle and magnesium to let it go flaccid – a simple physiological fact. We spend a lot of time flexing our muscles in the actions of being, laughing, blinking, and not a lot of time giving them what they need to relax. Some high-magnesium foods are oats, dates, nuts, figs, milk, seafood, molasses, seeds, wheat germ, and other whole grains. Congrats if you are eating all of those! Here is the list of things that can deplete you of magnesium: stress, stomach upset, antibiotics, and oral contraceptives. Whoops, maybe you are experiencing or using all of the above. Magnesium is a mineral that is hard to extract from food (it's a rock after all).

The reasons we are magnesium depleted are threefold: we need more than we get from our diet, our plants contain less than we need, and our digestion isn't working so as to extract whatever is there. So, the tweak this week is to get more magnesium into your diet.

An example of optimum daily magnesium intake might include one cup of yogurt, one cup of oatmeal, five almonds, five ounces of fish, and one cup of warm milk (before bed). It will take a while to build up your magnesium stores, so keep up this regime for several weeks. Even with the perfect number of servings of food sources it helps to have a little magic boost. Supplementing with 100 milligrams of magnesium immediately before bed can do wonders. Fairly quickly, the body takes this mineral, given just when you need it the most, and uses it to its own advantage.

SLEEP-NUT COOKIES

Here is an evening snack to be eaten two or three hours before bed that will increase your magnesium level in the tastiest way possible and soothe you into slumber. Two cookies and one cup of milk is an excellent high-magnesium snack that's less than 300 calories.

	Ingredients	*Benefits*
2 cups	any combo of all-natural peanut butter and/or almond butter	magnesium for muscles
¼ cup	molasses	iron for blood
¼ cup	honey	mineral-containing sweetener
1	egg	protein for muscles
3–6 tbsp	whole-wheat flour (amount depends upon the grind of the nuts)	fibre for colon health

Combine all ingredients except flour in a bowl and mix with a spatula. Sprinkle in 1 tbsp of flour at a time until dough comes together and is quite thick and less sticky. Use your hands to roll into 36 small balls and place onto a baking sheet. Press with a fork. Bake at 350°F for 8–10 minutes. The cookies should be a little soft in the middle; they will harden as they cool.

Preparation time: 10 minute Servings: 36 cookies (2 cookies per serving)

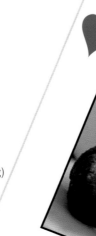

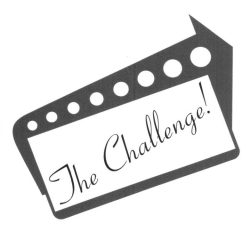

The Challenge!

GIVEN HOW HELPFUL MAGNESIUM is in managing stress by helping muscles relax and ameliorating heart disease, I often recommend it as a supplement to my clients. Investigate magnesium supplements; they are available online, and in drugstores, grocery stores, and health food stores. No need to spend a lot of money (magnesium is way cheaper than sleeping pills!). There is even a gel that is absorbed through the skin. Write down how much a good night's sleep will cost you per day.

PRICE OF MAGNESIUM SUPPLEMENT

$_____

QUANTITY

_____

COST PER DAY

$_____

JACK OF HEARTS

FISH: Go Fish

We need to eat more fish. That's the bottom line. Fish doesn't just protect our hearts. Studies have shown other health benefits, such as lowered risk of breast, colon, and prostate cancers as well as eye, brain, and joint health improvements. Fish contain oil that is rich in omega-3 fatty acids, which have anti-inflammatory effects. Studies have also shown improved symptoms in people suffering with mental and depressive disorders when they supplement with omega-3 from fish oil.

There is no consensus on specific dietary recommended intake of omega-3, but most experts suggest between 500 and 2,000 milligrams per day from all sources. As explored in other cards, we know we can get omega-3 from non-fish sources, such as eggs, and foods like flax and chia seeds, as well as from supplements. However, the most direct route is to consume omega-3 from the kind of fat called DHA, which only comes from animal sources. And the best animal source is fish. Canada's current recommendations are a mere two or three servings of fish per week, which seeks to balance health benefits against the risks from mercury and other pollutants found in fish. The Institute of Medicine assessed many studies looking at the risks and benefits of partaking from the sea and it makes the recommendation that children under 12 or women who are pregnant or wishing to become

pregnant can safely consume up to 12 ounces per week (including six ounces of canned tuna). Other than that limitation, the benefits of eating fish outweigh the risks of mercury contamination. If you are like most people who do not live on a seacoast, you are likely getting only one serving per week, if that, so how to get two more? And which seafood should you consume? The top three consumed in North America are tuna, salmon, and shrimp, so that's a good place to start.

TUNA: The Seven of Spades covered the first, cheapest, and most convenient way of eating fish: canned tuna, which is a moderate source of omega-3. Consuming one can per week of skipjack (sometimes called light, or flaked, tuna) will net less mercury than eating the larger, darker albacore (sometimes called chunk, or solid). Skipjack tuna is also cheaper. The other two servings should come from different oceans and different types of fish, to lower the risk of one toxin accumulating.

SALMON: Most people love salmon and it is an excellent source of omega-3. But which type should you choose? Remember that big exposé a few years back saying that farmed salmon had way more mercury than wild? There's more to the story. The "wild" salmon that was chosen for comparison was a type that isn't normally sold at the grocery store. It was so wild that most of us can't buy it. It also turns out that the feed was skewing the mercury numbers. Since then the farmed salmon industry has made careful strides to monitor the fish feed more closely and measure the contaminants better.

But it's farmed fish! Isn't that bad? Think of it this way: this planet has way too many people on it and we are all going to need to be fed. It would be utopia if we could all move to the farm, grow our own food, and fish in ponds that are spring-fed with pollutant-free crystal waters. The dilemma is that we know we need to consume more fish for our health, but the oceans are having trouble keeping up with our relentless demand. What are we to do? We need to count on farmers as we always have, and urge them to do their most conscientious job of getting food on our tables. *All* of our tables. If there is enough wild fish to go around without annihilating the species and/or habitat and you can find as well as afford it, go ahead. But don't avoid salmon simply because you are afraid of the mercury bogey man.

SHRIMP: This popular shellfish has a moderate omega-3 rating but it is the number one seafood on the market. Some fear that it has too much cholesterol for weekly consumption but a serving of shrimp per week has little or no negative impact upon our cholesterol levels and it is an otherwise lean, omega-3 containing protein. The World Wildlife Fund is currently working with the shrimp farming industry to create better practices; so if you are going to buy shrimp, buy American for now until the rest of the world gets on board.

The healthiest fish for us (and for the planet) are the smaller fish. Sadly these are used as bait or "chum" and include delicious species like herring and sardines. Both weigh in with as much, if not more, omega-3 as salmon and are cheap and plentiful. The bonus of eating these fish is that it helps to create a more sustainable fishing industry and healthier oceans for us and the planet. You can easily buy a $2 can of either and the recipe below for serving them fresh will wow your next dinner party or brunch.

BARBECUED SMALL FISH

This recipe uses smelts, herring, or sardines. You may need to go to a fish market to find these smaller fish, but it's worth the effort as their sweet, delicate meat cooks in mere minutes. Purchase them cleaned. Eating them is simple: just slide your fork over one side to pull off the flesh, thus exposing the skeleton, which can be lifted away whole.

Ingredients

		Benefits
1–1½ lb	small fish	sustainable omega-3 source
1	lemon, sliced	enhances bile for digestion
2 tbsp	capers	rutin; promotes healthy blood vessels
¼ cup	fresh dill (or 1 tbsp dried)	trace vanadium; lowers blood pressure
4–6 dashes	hot sauce	capsaicin; boosts metabolism

Place fish in a glass casserole dish or lasagna pan. Slice lemons very thinly and lay on top of fish. Sprinkle capers and dill over fish and splash with hot sauce. Bake in 425°F oven or on barbecue for 6–8 minutes. Season at the table with sea salt or Sea(soning) Mix (recipe on page 118) and pepper.

Preparation time: 4 minutes Servings: 4

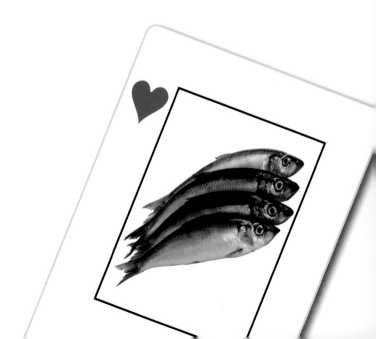

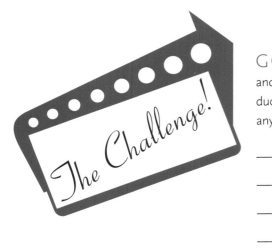
The Challenge!

GO ONLINE AND TYPE in the phrase "sustainable fish" and read at least one article. Look for sites that are not sponsored by fish producers but by government organizations or wildlife foundations. Write down any notes below:

_____
_____
_____
_____
_____
_____
_____
_____
_____
_____
_____
_____
_____
_____

TEN OF HEARTS

RED MEAT: Have your steak and eat it too!

———

There is no longer any doubt that we need to reduce our consumption of red meat (which includes pork), and the reasons are mounting. Many experts (including one of the doctors at my practice) insist that we have to eat a completely plant-based diet if we want to avoid the major diseases that plague us. I like my steak or burger, once in a while, but I am serving less conventionally raised meat in my home. That's not a step for everyone, but I know that my loved ones count on me to lead the way.

Here is why our red meat consumption has to go down.

❶ IT'S TOO MUCH OF A BAD THING: Read any of the popular, conscientious food journalists and you'll find they all agree on a major point: conventionally raised animals live unpleasant, often cruel, lives in poor conditions and on feed that is either indigestible or insufficient. This practice turns out meat that is not good for us (cancer, diabetes, heart disease) *and* we eat too much of it. The key issue is that the grain fed to cows (rather than their natural food, grass) gives their meat more of the bad saturated fat and less of the good omega-3 fat.

❷ THE NEGATIVE IMPACT UPON OUR PLANET AND ITS PEOPLE OF RAISING COWS FOR MEAT OR DAIRY IS ENORMOUS. Cattle excrete large quantities of methane gas, which is one of the greenhouse gases affecting our atmosphere. Plus, if we fed all that grain to people instead of cows (who turn it into concentrated protein for us at great expense), we would have fewer, if any, hungry people in the world. When I consider what to put on my plate, this misuse of resources does factor into my decision.

❸ WHEN COLD PROTEIN HITS HOT GRILLS OR PANS, A CHEMICAL REACTION CREATES TWO MUTAGENS: heterocyclic amines (HCAs) and polycyclic aromatic hydrocarbons (PAHs). When ingested, these molecules cause changes to DNA that can lead to cancer. Beef is the biggest offender, chicken and fish less so.

There are ways to eat meat and, with a little shift, make a huge difference in your health, and that of the planet and its animals.

- Statistics are showing that Canadians are reducing consumption of beef, processed meats, and pork, and moving toward chicken and fish. This is a good trend. The recommendation is to indulge in meat no more than once per week, and the more often you replace any meat with poultry, fish, beans, nuts, or soy for protein, the greater the impact on your health.
- Switch from beef to lamb once in a while, too. It is easier to find and cheaper to buy grass-fed lamb than grass-fed beef. Buying a frozen lamb leg and roasting the whole thing can get you Sunday dinner for four, a few sandwiches for lunches and some soup from the bone for $20. When you want your steak or burger, spend more on a slightly smaller portion of organic, or at least grass-fed, beef. Because you are eating less beef less often, you can afford to indulge in better quality.
- Learn how to cook meat to reduce the formation of the bad HCAs and PAHs. Simply switch up your cooking method to any style that keeps the meat wet, such as braising, stewing, and roasting at lower temperatures. And if you grill, rub or marinate the meat beforehand. Even a quick dip or rub with any combo spices/oil/acid before the meat hits the flames will reduce the HCAs and PAHs .

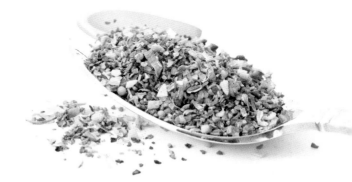

LOW-SODIUM, HIGH-FLAVOUR, PROTEIN-PROTECTIVE SPICE RUB

This rub can be used on any meat, chicken, or fish before you barbecue. The antioxidants in the herbs will help you fight off the HCAs and PAHs, and the quick addition of oil and vinegar will help protect the meat from creating them in the first place. This recipe makes a large batch that will keep in the spice cupboard for months.

	Ingredients	*Benefits*
1 tbsp	kosher salt	larger grain delivers more salt flavour so you can use less
1 tbsp	freshly ground black pepper	capsaicin; revs metabolism
1 tsp	paprika	antioxidants
1 tsp	dill seed	helps digestion
2 tsp	mustard seed	isothiocyanates; anticarcinogenic
2 tbsp	dried rosemary	acetylcholine; protects neurotransmitters
1 tbsp	dried onion flakes	sulphur; blood thinner
1 tsp	dried minced garlic	allicin; reduces cholesterol
1 tsp	garlic powder	traditional cough expectorant
¼–½ tsp	crushed red pepper	creates feeling of satiety
1 tsp	onion powder	blood-thinning potential

Use approximately ½ tsp per portion (4–5 oz) of meat. Rub into meat, along with ½ tsp grapeseed oil and ½ tsp of any vinegar or lemon juice. Heat grill to maximum; turn it down just before you add the meat and cook over medium heat until cooked through.

Preparation time: 6 minutes Servings: 24 (½ teaspoon each)

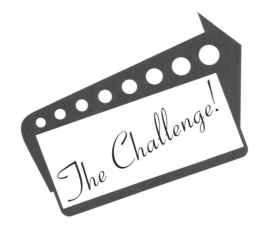

The Challenge!

HOW MUCH DO YOU spend on beef, pork, and processed meats each week? Take a look at an old grocery bill and write the amount here: $ _____

How much could you save if you ate these products only once per week? $ _____

What is the cost per pound of either grass-fed beef or lamb at your local grocery store? $ _____

Did you save enough to treat your family to a better, safer, healthier, and greener cut?

NINE OF HEARTS

CHEESE: A condiment, not a meal

One of the hardest things about going to my book club is avoiding the cheese platter. Throughout our discussion, I eye the yummy, beckoning cheeses sitting on the coffee table. Sometimes they call my name so loud, particularly the blue cheese and its siren song, that I am not able to focus on the conversation.

Before dealing with cheese, a note about milk and dairy products in general. Some people can't digest or tolerate milk and dairy products, and the only way to know if you're one of those people is to cut them out of your diet and see if you feel better. I am not going to "whey" in on the debate about whether humans are meant to drink milk, but I will address its impact on our overall health. Milk is caloric and contains fat (unless you go fat-free), but in return it does provide protein, calcium, and some other minerals.

Switching to organic milk is beneficial, for the simple reason that you avoid some of the pesticides, toxins, and hormone residues that are consumed by cows through commercial feed. Even if you remove the fat, as in skim milk, the residues remain. Avoiding consumption of these minute, but accumulating, chemicals is a good idea.

But back to my book club. I know I need to avoid my beloved cheese platter for three reasons:

❶ FAT. Many cheeses are so high in saturated fat that they make steak look like diet food. The body needs very little saturated fat and it may be contributing to our LDL cholesterol. What do you think "triple cream" brie means? It means that the cheese is 70 to 75 percent fat, which is as close to butter as a knife can get! We wouldn't dream of scooping up hunks and wedges of butter to load onto our cracker. Even the most common, innocuous cheese, cheddar, is about 30 to 33 percent milk fat.

❷ LACK OF NUTRIENTS PER CALORIE. Cheese is extremely caloric and costly for what it delivers on nutrients. Unless it is a low-fat cheese, it contains as much fat as protein or more. The benefits like calcium, potassium, and magnesium that cheese delivers can be obtained in less damaging foods.

❸ SALT. The process of making cheese requires a significant amount of sodium. For instance, one cup of low-fat cottage cheese contains about half a day's worth of salt. Four small squares of cheddar, ditto. Salt and fat are much of what makes cheese so enticing, why we crave it, and how it lures us into eating more.

So what's a girl to do? I can't avoid book club, cocktail parties, and baby showers forever! The trick is to stop thinking of cheese as a way of eating protein. It does have protein but the cost in calories, sodium, and saturated fat isn't worth it.

- Suss out cheeses like one made in the Netherlands called Cantenaar, which has 40 percent less fat and 25 percent less salt than other cheeses. It tastes a bit like Gouda but is not at all like the rubbery low-fat alternative cheeses available, which are also high in salt.

- Cheeses made with goat's milk are naturally lower in fat and ridiculously tasty. Sodium varies by brand so choose one that is less than 200 milligrams per 50-gram serving.

- Mitigate the amount of cheese per mouthful. Instead of having a hunk of cheese on a salty cracker, think about having a sliver of cheese on an apple slice or celery stick. You'll eliminate the calories and salt from the cracker, add nutrients and fibre with the fruit, and consume less fat.

GOAT CHEESE AND ARTICHOKE SPREAD

When you are going to a party, bringing a spread that is at least half water and vegetables but that also sports a cheese moniker is a great idea. Eat your own spread first and don't make it too often at home. Turn to this when you need to look away from the blue and the Camembert.

Ingredients

1 cup	marinated artichoke hearts, drained	potassium for homeostasis*
¾ cup	chèvre cheese	lower-fat dairy
¼ tsp	mustard	high-antioxidant flavouring
1 tsp	herbes de Provence	trace minerals
¼ tsp	garlic powder	antibacterial
2 tbsp	nutritional or flaked yeast	probiotic; for bowel health
¼ cup	slivered almonds	calcium; for bone health

Benefits heads the third column.

Use a mini-chopper or hand blender to purée all ingredients except almonds. Spread into a crock or serving dish and top with almonds. Can be served warm or cold. To warm, place in 350°F oven for 15–20 minutes. Serve with celery sticks and whole-grain, low-sodium crackers.

Preparation time: **6 minutes** Servings: **12**

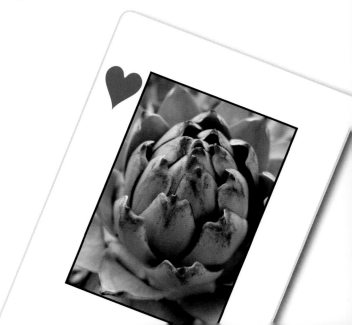

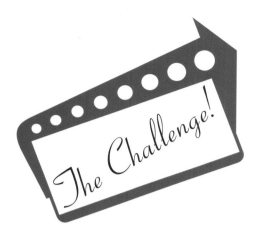

The Challenge!

NEXT TIME YOU ARE at an event that is cheesy, have a strategy. Sit as far away from the cheese tray as you can. Drink a glass of water before you start in on the cheese. Tell yourself that you will have some cheese but only after you are as full of vegetables and fruit as you could possibly be. Be the one who brings the veg and be the one who leaves without a heavy heart (literally and figuratively).

EIGHT OF HEARTS

FAT: Big fat confusion

———————

Almost every food has a little bit of fat in it with the exception of some fruits and vegetables. And we've been told that fats fall into two clear-cut categories, good and bad, right? But it isn't really that simple.

We need fat in our diet to make our hormones, insulate our bodies, and absorb fat-soluble vitamins. We do know that we need *some* saturated fat, which comes from foods, mostly animal sources, like meat and cheese, but also from plant sources, like coconut and palm. We also know that the better fats are the ones that are liquid at room temperature. But answering the questions How much? And from what? can be a minefield.

For heart health we need between 20 and 30 percent of the calories we consume each day to come from fats, as long as we can do that without gaining weight. But unless you are a human calculator this information isn't of much use. In order to ace your health you need to think about what you are getting *with* that fat. For instance, extra virgin olive oil is cold pressed and has not been heat- or chemically processed so it still has its health-promoting polyphenols

intact. It may be the polyphenols that are doing the cholesterol-lowering, heart-protecting, cancer-preventing, skin-brightening heavy work. Compare the fat in two tablespoons of olive oil to that overheated canola oil in a small McDonald's fries. They each have about 200 calories, but one is much better than the other. (And, no, it's not the fries.)

Deep frying kills any polyphenols that may have been in the canola oil to begin with, so there goes your benefit, now there's just calories. The rest of the story is how that fat was processed before it even hit the heat in the deep fryer. Many fast-food restaurants have removed trans fats, yes, but the substitute oils were likely heat- and chemically treated to extract the fat from the seed even before they went into the deep fryer. When this oil is reheated at high temperatures, the molecules twist into a form that may be carcinogenic. You can see why I say, "Nothing deep fried, ever." In the interest of full disclosure: you may have seen me at the pub last week eating *six* of my friend's fries, but I gave my body the extra nutrients from some collard greens to help clean up the damage.

So the question becomes, what fats are worth eating given their caloric heft? It's that "pull its weight" perspective again. If it is going into your body, it had better be doing more than just filling you up and tasting yummy, it has to *add* something.

SATURATED FATS

Milk fats: You already know about red meat and cheese and how to get the most of the good that they have to offer while mitigating the bad. These limits benefit your heart health in two ways: by reducing the fats in your blood and helping you manage your weight. Milk has its place but you want the most calcium, vitamin D, and magnesium for your glass with the least fat and calories. Skim milk has the same number of nutrients with none of the fat, so with each percentage of fat you go up, you are increasing *only* calories. You can get calcium from other sources (almonds, broccoli, and soy and rice drinks) that is equally, if not more, absorbable, and they may be lower in calories.

Time to wade in to the butter versus margarine debate: the answer is, go for butter. Margarine is made from oils that have been heated, treated, and depleted, as described above. The newer versions may no longer have trans fats but neither do the fries, remember? One teaspoon of either butter or margarine has exactly the same number of calories but butter is a fat that the body can digest and recognize as food. Plus, according to recent investigation it appears that butter's effect on cholesterol levels is exactly neutral; it neither raises nor lowers cholesterol. Regardless of which you choose, try to have no more than about a tablespoon per day, balancing this fat intake with whatever else you consume that day.

Medium-chain triglycerides: The middle child in the fat family is coconut oil. Unfortunately, if you lived through the eighties, you heard that coconut milk, oils, and meat are just as bad for you as saturated fats, but that's not completely true. Coconut oil *that has not been hydrogenated* is one of the better oils to be used in cooking. Its molecules can handle the heat without becoming twisted and toxic. Plus, coconut milk is one of the medium-chain triglycerides, which are shorter and easier to absorb than the longer chains. So a yummy coconut milk Thai green curry once in a while, while caloric, is also pretty good for you.

UNSATURATED FATS

You want most of your fat intake to come from whole-food, unheated, unsaturated sources. These fats are the ones that consistently show up as cardio-protective because they either lower cholesterol or they come with other gifts like antioxidants, vitamins, and minerals. Information on the benefits of the fats from nuts and seeds is sprinkled throughout the book so I won't belabour that point.

Just remember that they are best for you in their natural, unheated, unsalted state, particularly hemp seeds, the only commonly used seed that contains GLA, a crucial, hormone-regulating fat that is rare in other foods.

Oils (extra virgin olive oil for salads and grapeseed for higher temperature cooking): Grapeseed oil's temperature can be raised quite high before it begins to smoke so it is less damaged by the heat. It also may help prevent the oxidation of cholesterol. This oxidation is what does the damage to the cardiovascular system, and there is some evidence that the antioxidants in grape seeds help protect blood vessel damage that occurs with high blood pressure. But there is one caveat: your brand must be minimally processed and you must heat it in a specific manner. You want to heat your pan *first* to medium or high heat without any oil in it. Have your ingredients ready to go in before you add the oil and add the food as quickly as you can after you add the oil. This will prevent sticking, preserve the oil, and give a better colour and texture to your food. What's not to like? Extra virgin olive oil is an excellent source of unsaturated fats. This is only true if it is cold pressed and served raw and unheated.

Avocados: Avocados are loaded with good (monounsaturated) fat. Again, during the fat-phobic 1980s people were scared off avocados by the fact that they have *loads* of calories, but with these you get *loads* of super-nutrients. Avocados are normally eaten raw so you are getting the good fat at its peak. They also contain potassium to regulate blood pressure and the nutrient folate for heart health. Adding some avocado to your salad makes the fat-soluble vitamins more available to your body.

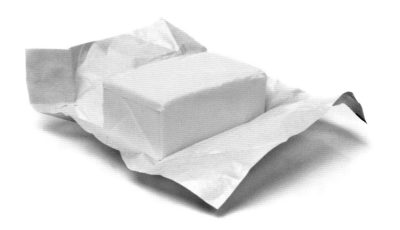

VS.

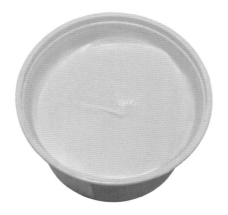

CREAMY AVOCADO DRESSING

Feel free to use commercial pesto as long as it contains only extra virgin olive oil.

Ingredients		*Benefits*
¼	ripe avocado	folic acid, fibre, and good fat
1 tbsp	pesto	chlorophyll; for liver function
pinch	sea salt (or herbal salt mix)	higher minerals than table salt
1 tsp	garlic powder	antimicrobial; protects heart
1 tbsp	extra virgin olive oil	polyphenols; prevent heart disease
¼–½ cup	lime juice	vitamin C; antioxidant
¼–½ cup	water	

Use a hand blender or mini-chopper to blend all ingredients together. Store in a glass jar in the fridge for up to 10 days.

Preparation time: 5 minutes Servings: 10 to 12

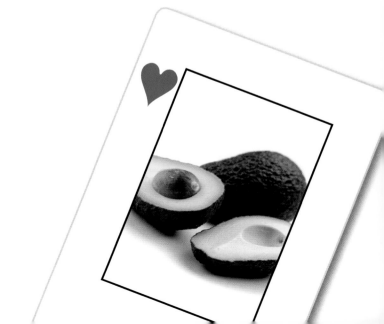

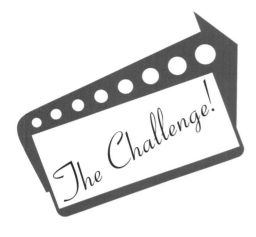

The Challenge!

LAST WEEK YOU KNEW less about fat than you do today. Within the categories below, list all of the fats that you ate last week that brought little else with them. These are the spare players who have got to go or at least must be sent to the bench more often.

Candy bars, cakes, and treats:

_____

Commercial salad dressings:

_____

Cooking oils other than grapeseed:

_____

Deep-fried foods:

_____

Over-heated olive oil:

_____

SEVEN OF HEARTS

SALT: Salty dog

We need salt in our diets, and too little can cause as much trouble as too much. Sodium works with potassium to regulate the fluid levels in each and every cell in our bodies. People usually pay attention to salt only when they have received the bad news that they have hypertension (high blood pressure), or they can't get their rings off their swollen fingers the morning after a bucket of movie theatre popcorn.

Excess salt (and too little potassium and other minerals) makes our bodies retain water, putting extra stress on blood vessels, which may, over time, make the heart have to work harder. That same effect is happening in every cell, including those little pouches under the eyes. (The more often salt-saturated blood pools and stretches the skin, the more permanent those pouches will be.) I can bust my husband for a salty lunch just by looking at him when he gets home at dinner. Still, we think mainly in terms of heart health when we think of a salty diet. Health Canada is among many groups around the world that have put a number on how much salt we should have and it's much lower than our national average of 3,100 milligrams per day (at least that's lower than the American estimate of 4,000 milligrams). Low-risk populations should have no more than 2,300 milligrams per day, higher-risk people (defined as anyone over 40 and anyone of African descent or with a previous diagnosis of high blood pressure) should have no more than 1,500 milligrams per day. We need only 500 milligrams to sustain the healthy electrolyte balance our nerves and muscles must have to function properly.

But to get the whole story, as usual, we need to look at what comes *with* the salt. One of the goals of this book is to provide easy methods to get your salt intake down to a reasonable amount. The simplest way to do so is to follow the DASH diet (Dietary Approaches to Stop Hypertension) created by the U.S. National Institutes of Health, which has been proven to do just that. DASH is nothing more than a sensible eating plan. The tune is familiar:

consume mostly fruits and vegetables, some low-fat dairy, whole grains and high fibre, fish at least twice per week, poultry for other protein, as well as beans, seeds, and nuts, and limit intake of red meat, salt, and sweets. However, given our dependence upon convenience foods that are salt loaded, following DASH can seem overwhelming.

The human taste for salt grows along with its consumption, so it can sneak up on you. The good news is that you quickly acclimatize when you switch back to a lower salt load and start tasting the real flavours of food again. Salt is cheap and acts as a preservative, so it bulks up manufactured food in a way that serves manufacturers, not consumers. There are now low-sodium versions of almost every food item imaginable and that's because we are buying more of them. Eating low-salt versions frees up some sodium space for the truly "worth it" foods.

The trick is to balance sodium intake with potassium and other minerals.

- Switch to sea salt. Table salt is 99 percent sodium chloride with some iodine added to prevent goitre, which is not really an issue today because we get so much table salt from processed foods. Sea salt is 95 to 98 percent sodium chloride and the remaining amount is trace minerals including potassium. These other minerals help the body process the sodium.
- Follow the Five of Spades crash course in label reading and reduce the "not worth it" sodium load.
- Salt foods after they are cooked. It takes twice as much salt to flavour a food from within as it does on top. The tongue wants to taste the salt, and when it comes first, as on the top of a cracker, we are more easily satisfied.
- Look for some of the commercially available sea salt and herb mixes. They are great at adding other flavours beyond salt. Rather than crystallized salt, flake salt or sel de mer is less dense by nature so you will get less sodium per pinch of flavour but it is pricier.
- Make the Sea(soning) Mix on the next page and keep it on the table.
- Give your palate a chance to adapt! Foods will taste a little bland for a week or so while you are reducing sodium, but it won't take long before you notice a broader range of delightful flavours.

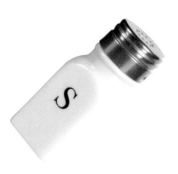

SEA(SONING) MIX

Use this seasoning by the pinchful at the end of cooking or to season at the table.
You can buy the ingredients in small amounts at bulk food stores.

Ingredients		*Benefits*
1 tbsp	sea salt, coarsely ground	dissolves slowly; saltiness lingers longer
1 tbsp	sea salt, finely ground	minerals, electrolyte balance
1 tbsp	poultry seasoning	carries salty flavour further
1 tsp	garlic powder	enhances flavour
1 tsp	dried thyme	antioxidant
1 tsp	cracked black pepper	enhances metabolism
¼ tsp	cayenne pepper	boosts flavour
2 tsp	red chili pepper flakes	creates feeling of satiety

Mix ingredients together. Put into a salt cellar or other serving container.
It takes a mere pinch or sprinkle to highly season any dish. Keep on the table for
diners to use to add taste to many dishes.

Preparation time: 1 minute Servings : 64 pinches (less than ¼ tsp)

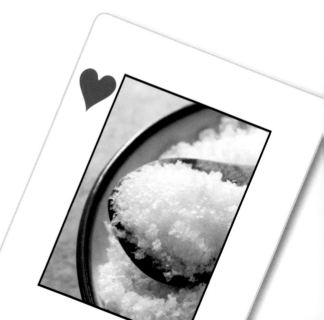

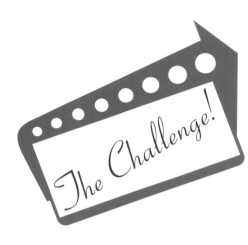
The Challenge!

ADD UP YOUR POTASSIUM foods for the day and work on eating more healthy high-potassium foods as you decrease the salt. (Watch your puffy eyes for any response!)

HIGH-POTASSIUM FOODS:

Dried fruits

Tomato paste

Baked potatoes

Bananas

Artichokes

Broccoli

Mushrooms

Fennel

Kiwi

Oranges

Prunes

Sardines

Yogurt

Chicken

Nuts

Beans (dried and boiled, or canned and well-rinsed)

Wheat germ

Cocoa powder

Molasses

SIX OF HEARTS

SOUP: Soup(er) trooper

Soup is soothing and tastes great, lightens the nasal congestion of a cold, is a low-calorie yet high-nutrient food, and is easy on the pocketbook. The trouble with most commercial soups is that the nutrients are watered down and the salt is ratcheted up. Broth should be semi-firm (like Jell-O) when it has enough protein and flavour in it, but many manufacturers fill up their products with water, cheap pasta, or other fillers as well as salt, rather than investing in real food.

For the purposes of heart health there are two reasons to eat soup: as an appetizer, it displaces the hunger for the more calorie-laden food that usually comes next and, as a main course, it can deliver a bunch of nutrition in one spoonful. Think about how much spinach cooks down. You can slip a whole bag of spinach into a broth and one spoonful delivers a powerful punch!

The Jack of Spades already convinced you that you need to eat more slowly. Hot, multi-textured soup, eaten with a spoon, forces you to slow down. Plus, it is soothing and warm and engages the senses.

Calorie displacement studies show that a bowl of broth or low-cal vegetable-based (rather than high-cal cream-based) soup eaten *before* a meal will cause the eater to compensate and uncon-sciously consume fewer calories during that meal. Soup does this even better than a salad or a glass of water. Removing a couple of hundred calories per day means losing a couple of pounds per month. Lightening the load that your heart needs to carry is a very important step in protecting it.

Making homemade chicken stock is as simple as keeping the bones from any cooked chicken and boiling them in a pot or slow cooker. The liquid pulls protein, calcium, and precious minerals from the bones. Once you have the (didn't cost you a dime!) stock, it can be filled with nourishing greens to create a high-protein, high-nutrient, low-calorie, low-sodium main course that will stand on its own. If there's a perfect food, soup is it.

SIMPLE HOMEMADE STOCK

Any time you eat chicken, save the bones and store them in the freezer until you get about six cups' worth, which is about one small carcass. Keep the stock frozen in one-cup portions to warm up whenever you want, or use it right away in this rich and tasty soup.

Ingredients

Amount	Ingredient	Benefits
6 cups	chicken bones (or the carcass from a roasted or store-bought cooked chicken)	protein
2	unpeeled onions, halved	allicin; reduces cholesterol
2	garlic cloves, smashed	enhance immunity
2	carrots, quartered	beta carotene for eyes
1 tbsp	vinegar	draws out calcium from chicken bones

Half-fill a slow cooker or large pot with cold water and add bones, onions, garlic cloves, and carrots. Add vinegar and stir. Turn slow cooker on high for 6–8 hours, or if cooking on stovetop bring to a boil, turn down to a simmer, and cook for 2–3 hours. Strain through a sieve and discard bones and scraps. Store stock in fridge for up to 5 days or in freezer up to 8 weeks. Use as a base for homemade soups, like Serious Green Soup.

Preparation time: 10 minutes + simmer time Servings: 8 to 10

SERIOUS GREEN SOUP

Ingredients   *Benefits*

8–10 cups	homemade chicken stock	low-sodium, high-mineral
1	garlic bulb	enhances immunity
1 tbsp	dried onion (or chopped fresh)	controls cholesterol
1 tsp	dried thyme	micronutrients; prevent cancer
1 tsp	dried basil	micronutrients; prevent cancer
2 cups	frozen peas	fibre; lowers cholesterol
4	small zucchini, chopped	lutein; for eye health
4 cups	baby spinach	folate; repairs cells
	Sea(soning) Mix and pepper, to taste	enhances digestion
28-oz can	lupini or other beans (optional)	earth-friendly protein
1 tbsp	Parmesan cheese	calcium for teeth

Pour chicken stock into a large pot and add bulb of garlic and the onion. Bring to a boil, then simmer for 20–30 minutes. Use a slotted spoon to pluck out garlic and onion; add thyme, basil, peas, and diced zucchini. Simmer for 5 minutes. Squeeze softened boiled garlic cloves into soup. Stir in spinach and simmer 1–3 minutes, until leaves are barely cooked. Taste and add Sea(soning) Mix (see page 118) and pepper as needed. Serve as is, or purée with a hand wand or in a blender if you prefer a creamier soup. To make a heartier meal, stir in (drained) beans and top with a tablespoon of Parmesan cheese.

Preparation time: 15 minutes Servings: 8

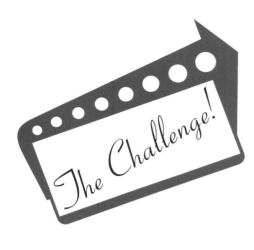

START EACH SUPPER MEAL this week with a bowl of soup. Note what kind of soup you had and whether you felt less hungry during and after the meal. Did your pants feel a little looser at the end of the week?

	WHAT KIND OF SOUP I ATE	HOW I FELT
MONDAY		
TUESDAY		
WEDNESDAY		
THURSDAY		
FRIDAY		
SATURDAY		
SUNDAY		

FIVE OF HEARTS

––––––––––

You know the drill, you've been doing it, or watching people do it, for years: "Sauce on the side, please." The sauces in restaurant and frozen foods are intended to make the dish shiny and to have a nice "mouth feel," which means more butter or other fats than you care to think about. It is a good idea when you are dining out to order a grilled dish and have the sauce on the side. And when you are at home, you can create incredible sauces without the extra fats.

The easiest one to make is a demi-glace. It is made from homemade stock (like the stock from the Six of Hearts) that is simply boiled down. One cup of stock will reduce to about three or four tablespoons of the best-tasting, mouth-feeling, restaurant-standard sauce that will make you the envy of your fellow chefs. On its own it's delish and contains every bit as much protein and minerals as the stock, minus the water. A tablespoonful over grilled or baked chicken or fish is wonderful. Make your steak sing by cooking some mushrooms with garlic and stirring them into the demi-glace.

Or you can make a creamy sauce for pasta or protein out of yogurt (recipe on page 126). You will consume some fat but nothing like what's in

a butter-based sauce. You will also gain the benefits of the calcium and protein in the yogurt but not, unfortunately, the probiotics. These live enzymes do not survive heating.

Tomato sauces are equally healthy if you make sure that you choose canned salt-free tomatoes and don't add salt to your sauce. My favourite way to make tomato sauce is to buy two to three pounds of beef bones for peanuts at the grocery store and brown them in a large pot. Then I add two cloves of minced garlic and one 28-ounce can of crushed tomatoes and let it simmer all day. Once the bones give up their marrow to the sauce, they can be scraped off and given to the dog. The flavour comes from the marrow, which is a good fat, rather than from the beef muscle protein (ground beef or cuts of meat), which contains mostly saturated fat. Using a few bones rather than a load of ground beef means that the sauce is lower in calories. This sauce is as good with beans or on pasta as it is on chicken breasts or grilled fish.

While I am on the topic of sauces, I may as well cover condiments, which many mistake for sauces. For everyday eating, mustard is your go-to condiment. It is made from nutritious, anti-inflammatory mustard seeds, is usually coloured with turmeric (a high-antioxidant spice), and rarely contains sugar. By comparison, mayonnaise, even the low-fat versions, is sometimes made with real eggs but is mostly just heated fats with lots of salt and sugar. One tablespoon of low-fat mayo can cost you 50 calories and five grams of bad fats. Better to skip it as often as you can.

Somewhere in between mustard and mayo are ketchup and relish. They are usually low in fat but high in sugar and they do have some, albeit cooked and depleted, vegetable in them. Try using only a teaspoon at a time and amping up the mustard. The same goes for barbecue sauce. In order to make wise decisions on which bottled sauce to use for easy meals, you need to employ your label-reading skills. I particularly like some of the Indian curry kits. They allow me to make a quick meal that is full of flavour and one that I wouldn't be able to create on my own quickly. The better ones contain real food, like tomatoes, onions, butter, and spices, rather than oils or gums or thickeners. The trick is to stretch them as far as they will go. If it says to add four chicken breasts, add six and a cup or two of frozen peas, plus some spinach. These steps will volumize the nutrients and dilute the fat and salt over more portions. Any leftovers can be frozen for a second meal – bonus!

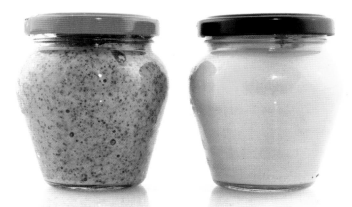

CREAMY YOGURT SAUCE

Simply switching up the herbs or adding mushrooms can entirely change the flavour of this versatile sauce. Use it as a pseudo–Alfredo or to top baked chicken or fish. Do not boil! The sauce will break down if overheated, so bring it just to the brink then turn down the heat.

Ingredients

		Benefits
1 tsp	butter	neutral effect on cholesterol
½	onion, finely chopped	sulphur; for heart health
1 tbsp	arrowroot powder or cornstarch ✳	fibre; aids digestion
1 cup	yogurt, plain	calcium and magnesium; for muscle control
¼ cup	dry white table wine	antioxidants; for heart health
½ cup	homemade chicken stock	sodium-free
1 tsp	dried thyme or marjoram	trace minerals; build muscle
pinch	Sea(soning) Mix	low in sodium

Warm a skillet over medium-high heat. Stir in butter and cook just long enough to allow it to brown ever so slightly. Stir in onion and allow to fully cook for 6–8 minutes, stirring often. Mix arrowroot powder into yogurt and let stand at room temperature for a few minutes. Set aside. Into the skillet, pour the wine and chicken stock, and add the thyme Seasoning Mix and boil for 2–4 minutes. Turn temperature down to medium-low and whisk in yogurt. Allow mixture to warm through for about 5 minutes.

OPTIONS:

- Change thyme to basil and stir in tomatoes and garlic at the end for a rosé sauce.
- Cook mushrooms separately and stir in with some rosemary at the end.
- Add apples and grated ginger to the wine and broth mix.
- Add ¼ cup grated Parmesan cheese and 1 tbsp of nutritional yeast for a cheesy sauce.

✳ Note: Arrowroot powder is a much better thickener than cornstarch, but it can be hard to find outside of health food stores. It is a good fibre that is easier to digest.

Preparation time: **20 minutes** Servings: **4**

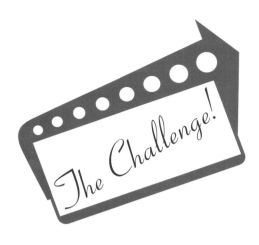

The Challenge!

YOUR CHALLENGE THIS WEEK is to tell someone else what sauce is all about. Share what you know in the gentlest way possible and, whatever you do, don't pass on your knowledge while they are eating anything on the "bad" list! Ask this person to tell you what sauces he or she eats regularly and write them down here, along with your own information. Then have that person over for dinner and serve the Creamy Yogurt Sauce.

	MY PAL	M E
BUTTER- OR OIL-BASED SAUCE		
CREAM SAUCE (MAC AND CHEESE, ALFREDO . . .)		
TOMATO SAUCE WITH MEAT		
MUSTARD		
MAYONNAISE		
OTHER CONDIMENTS		

FOUR OF HEARTS

ALCOHOL: Drinking buddy or arch rival?

I am often asked about alcohol and its place in a healthy diet. Sometimes the question is whispered with embarrassment, sometimes shouted with pride but always with confusion about whether, when, what, and how much to drink. It is no wonder we are confused: there is conflicting evidence simply because people aren't test tubes and we never drink alcohol in its isolated form. The answer is one of informed personal choice.

Scientific evidence confirms that there are more downsides than upsides to drinking alcohol, so if you don't drink, don't start. Alcohol reduces the amount of calories from fat that you burn, so if you are working your tail off at the gym to lose five pounds, the worst thing you can do is reward yourself with a beer! Alcohol also increases appetite and lowers inhibitions, causing your willpower to evaporate. This is dangerous because normally where there is beer, there is high-fat temptation. Alcohol also reduces testosterone levels and testosterone is the hormone you need to build and maintain muscle. All good reasons to abstain.

However, there is some evidence that one drink per day for women and two drinks per day for men is cardio-protective. No one is quite sure how alcohol protects the heart (yet!), but

theories range from its effect on the antioxidants in other foods to its ability to moderate our stress levels. Red wine comes with the most antioxidant power, and drinking alcohol along with high-antioxidant fruits or fruit juices does enhance their positive effects. The proviso is that "moderation" may mean consuæming less than you are accustomed to. So provided that your alcoholic intake doesn't outpace the number of calories burned each day, enjoying a glass or two may provide benefits. Plus, it is way more fun.

Here is the caveat: the liver is the organ doing all the work in metabolizing the alcohol and its effectiveness is based upon *its* health. We can protect the liver by eliminating the other toxins that it would otherwise have to process (which is what *Ace Your Health* is doing every week!): a high-fat diet, and inhalants like air fresheners, household cleaners, and petrochemical fumes. I'd rather avoid these things as much as possible and enjoy my wine, thanks. (And don't even think of taking an acetaminophen tablet to help recover from or prevent your hangover; the combination creates an enzymatic mash-up that can have disastrous effects on your liver.)

If you are going to consume alcohol, it is best to drink on a full stomach, which will slow down absorption and buy some time for your liver. Because fats empty from the stomach most slowly, it is best to have some of the good fats from an omega-3 source working for you while you drink. A simple tip stolen from a doctor I work with is to take a fish oil capsule before drinking. This is an easy magic bullet that helps to slow alcohol absorption and protects the liver, joints, and brain.

All things considered, if you are trying to lose weight, avoid alcohol. Give your liver 6 or 12 weeks to process that fat loss. Avoiding alcohol will also give you a head start by reducing calories, which will get you where you want to go faster, and getting there faster will give you more will power. Once you are at your goal weight, make an informed choice.

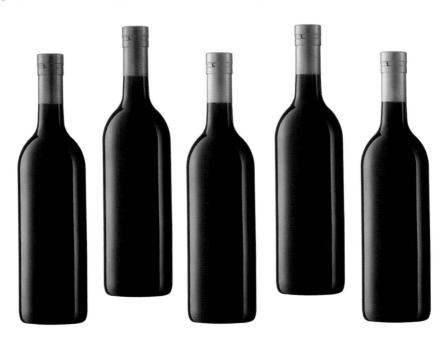

CANE AND ABLE

My husband and I set out to create the most potent antioxidant mixed drink we could concoct. We went with this combination of pomegranate juice sweetened with cane sugar (which has crucial trace minerals; see Nine of Clubs), vodka, and a few berries as garnish. The result is tasty and strong, which led our friends to rename the combo "Cane and Dis-Abled." We learned to drink a little less the next time. Scale up (on *all* ingredients) and make a whole pitcher for the crew.

	Ingredients	*Benefits*
3 oz	pure, unsweetened pomegranate juice	high in antioxidants/low in sugar
1–2 tsp	pure cane sugar	trace minerals; aid digestion
1–1¼ oz	vodka	enhances antioxidant uptake
3–5	ice cubes	water; aids liver function
3	berries (cranberries, blackberries, blueberries, or raspberries) for garnish	fibre and antioxidants

Stir together pomegranate juice, cane sugar, and vodka until sugar dissolves.
Pour over ice cubes. This mixture can be strained and served martini-style or topped with soda water and served in a highball glass. Garnish with berries.

Preparation time: 5 minutes Servings: 1 drink

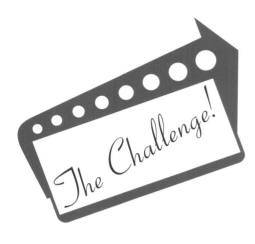
The Challenge!

BE A MIXOLOGIST. CREATE a beverage that is high in fruit or vegetables and so contains some fibre. It should stand alone as a "virgin" beverage that is low in calories without using artificial sweeteners. The addition of a moderate amount of alcohol will enhance the uptake of nutrients.

Name of my drink: _____

Serves: _____

Ingredients: _____

_____

Method: _____

_____

_____

_____ ounces fruit or vegetable juice

_____ ounces alcohol (no more than 1.25 ounces per drink)

_____ fruits or vegetables for garnish

_____ ice or sparkling water

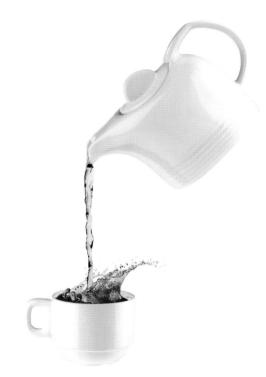

THREE OF HEARTS

TEA: It's the royal beverage for a reason

As I explained in the Queen of Spades, tea is a beverage you would be wise to include in your regimen, so a short course on the *Camellia sinensis* (aka tea) leaf is in order. All true teas are made from the same leaf; white, green, and black teas are simply treated differently at and after picking to create their different flavours and colours.

Black tea is most commonly used in orange pekoe teabags, which contain the dust and broken bits left over after the full leaves are packed off to use in finer brews. White tea is picked earlier and is rarer, and is the highest in antioxidants because it is processed least. Green tea, which includes oolong and jasmine, shows the most promise for its health benefits. In particular, it is the high content of EGCG (or epigallocatechin gallate for short!), and its positive effect on cancer cells. The amount of time that the leaf ferments creates the different teas. Green tea ferments the least, oolong is semi-fermented, and black tea ferments the longest. This is why it nets the heartiest true tea flavour, to stand up to adding milk and sugar. All teas deserve a splash in your cup.

The evidence on tea's health benefits continues

to mount. Tea has been shown to protect your teeth and your heart. One recent study showed a definitive link between tea drinking and reducing plaque in the arteries, which in turn has a positive effect on cardiovascular health.

True tea is made from *Camellia sinensis*; the other drinks that we often call "teas" are more appropriately called tisanes and are made from herbs, bushes, and berries. My favourite is rooibos, which originates in South Africa (*rooibos* means "red bush" in Afrikaans). Commercial tea companies have jumped on the bandwagon and rooibos is now widely available. Although it is less studied than "regular" tea, the news is encouraging. Rooibos is high in antioxidants, low in the flavour-enhancing but anti-nutrient tannins and contains no caffeine, which makes it a perfect stand-in when green or black tea isn't on offer, or when you're trying to cut down on caffeine or avoid oxalic acid (which contributes to kidney stones), or during pregnancy. It is strong and dark enough to fool you into believing that it is the real thing.

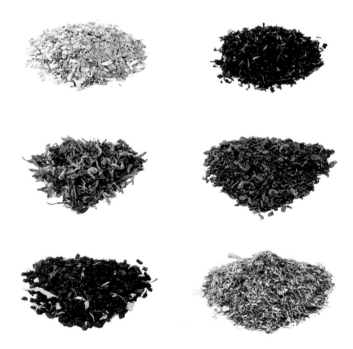

TEA-STEEPED PORK TENDERLOIN

Any tea will do in this recipe: the infusion of the flavours will work equally well with plain old orange pekoe teabags or rooibos. If serving for dinner and/or there are caffeine-sensitive people at the table, rooibos is the better choice.

	Ingredients	*Benefits*
2 ½ cups	boiling water	aids kidney function
3	rooibos teabags (or 3 tsp loose)	antispasmodic for stomach aches
1 tsp	allspice berries	eugenol (antiseptic)
1 tsp	juniper berries	volatile oils aid digestion
1 clove	garlic, crushed	scares away vampires
¼ cup	maple syrup	zinc for clear skin
2 tbsp	low-sodium soy sauce	trace minerals
2 lb	pork tenderloin	lean protein

In a large bowl, steep teabags with any combination of allspice and/or juniper berries until completely cooled. Stir in garlic, maple syrup, and soy sauce and pour into a resealable bag. Add pork tenderloin and store in fridge for 4–8 hours. Pour entire contents into a lasagna pan or casserole dish and place into a 425°F oven. Bake for 30–45 minutes until cooked through and some of the water has evaporated. Turn meat over once during cooking time. Slice and serve with brown rice and salad.

Preparation time: 5 minutes + marinating time Servings: 6

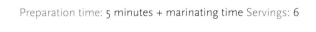

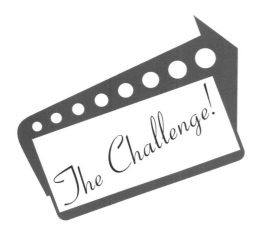

The Challenge!

TO BE SURE THAT you are getting the most out of your tea, brew whole, loose leaves. And loose leaves can make a cuppa that is cheaper and lower in caffeine. Here is how. Suss out a tea store or an online tea source. Ask a few questions (about origin, flavour, etc.) and sniff a few varieties, if you can. Find a green tea that you like and buy only 100 grams.

Use the same leaves all day and one teaspoon will go a long way. The first steep will contain most of the caffeine and each one after that will be weaker, until you are almost drinking water by the afternoon (see the Queen of Spades), which will help you get a good night's sleep.

To avoid much of the caffeine altogether, rinse the first steep of leaves with boiled water and discard after 20 seconds. A good portion of the caffeine will be rinsed down the drain, but the tea will still be strong in health benefits and flavour.

TWO OF HEARTS

BALANCING YOUR LIFE:
You are both passenger and conductor on this train

There are two ways that balance affects our hearts: one is in the metaphysical (work/home balance) sense and the other is in the physical (don't fall down) sense.

Metaphysical: First, let's look at work/home balance and the stress it can cause when it's out of whack. Many of us are pulled in different directions every day. By 9 a.m., I have already been a writer, food consultant, and nutritionist – and a mommy, wife, dog owner, and friend. Later in the day I may put on some lipstick and a smile to appear on television while trying to focus on not cutting my finger off as I impart nutritional information to my audience. At the end of the day, I get to fight city traffic while talking (illegally) to my mother on my cellphone and deciding what to make for dinner. My track-switching could employ an entire team of rail workers, but it is only *me, myself,* and *I* navigating this busy little engine.

On an unbalanced day I can feel my face flushing and my gut churning, signals that my body is out of balance. On a balanced day, I come home, pour a glass of wine, serve from the slow cooker with a smile, and regale my family with a hilarious incident from my day. I also have the time and patience to hear some of their joys, issues, and concerns. The cost of *not* switching tracks effectively is huge: our bodies wear out and gain weight with all the bottled-up stress. Our brain tells our adrenal glands to pump out adrenaline because we aren't coping. Adrenaline calls in its friends, the stress hormones, and their goal is to keep the body on high alert. Adrenaline and its friends tell the heart to beat faster, the lungs to work harder. This means the blood vessels to the skin and stomach are restricted, and they can't handle cleaning out waste via sweat or digestion right now. The trouble is that your body (not to mention your mind and your life) can only sustain this fight-or-flight reaction so often without suffering serious health consequences.

Balancing life's rigours well means knowing when to say no to lower-priority demands. Men tend to do this better than women. We all need to compartmentalize and delegate, say no, let it go, ask for help more often. Think of it as throwing unneeded baggage off your train as it is switching tracks. (With a little luck the rejects aren't something important, like a spouse or a pet!) Practising this manoeuvre teaches you how to make quick decisions about what to throw off your train and clarifies your priorities.

Physical: The body's sense of balance is simpler to understand but requires as much attention. Maintaining good posture makes the nerves that carry messages from the spine to the heart a lot more effective. If your physical balance is wonky, so are the messages from the body to the brain. Call up a mental image of a yogi in the tree pose: serenely standing on one leg with the other leg bent and the foot high up on the straight leg, hands in prayer position. It is virtually impossible to balance like this while track-switching. Every muscle in your body and your entire mind have to focus on one thing. Your eyes are open and gazing softly at a speck on the ground four or five feet away. (That speck is a metaphor for your life and the insignificance of its troubles to the workings of the universe, but never mind that right now.)

Both metaphysical and physical balance are mind games but with different rules; one moves quickly and the other very slowly. And both require clarity of purpose and a grounded sense of reality. The goal is to learn how to let your body know who is in charge, and tell your mind where to steer.

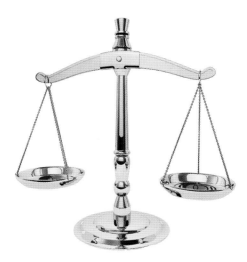

SEAFOOD SALSA

This easy recipe balances equal parts yogurt and salsa to create a delicious low-fat entrée.

Ingredients

		Benefits
1 ½ lb	salmon fillets (or other deboned fish)	omega-3 protein; reduces inflammation
¼ cup	plain yogurt	trace minerals for muscle control
¼ cup	salsa	antioxidant
1 bunch	asparagus	traditional arthritis treatment
¼ tsp	sea salt	trace minerals; aid digestion
1 tsp	dried oregano	antibacterial

Lay asparagus in a large, buttered baking dish and top with fish. Mix together yogurt, salsa, sea salt, and oregano and spread over fish. Bake, uncovered, at 400°F for 20–30 minutes, or until fish and asparagus are cooked through.

Preparation time: 5 minutes Servings: 4

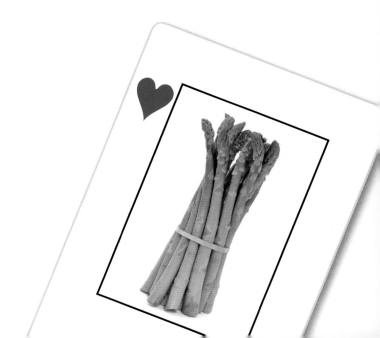

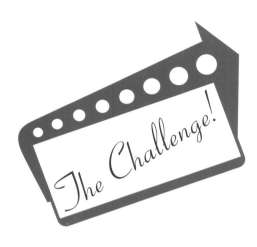
The Challenge!

THIS WEEK'S CHALLENGE IS to work toward that familiar yoga tree pose using a simple action that each of us does every day: putting on our socks and shoes.

Your current state of balance will determine your starting point. Jump into the list at whatever level you feel comfortable, and gradually build up to better balance. Work your way to the end as quickly or as slowly as suits you, but keep doing the exercise every day. Repeat a positive statement at every step, something like "I can balance my life" or "I can do better today in balancing my life" or "This is so stupid but maybe it will help me balance my life."

1. Use a wall to help you balance, standing up, while you pull on one sock at a time.
2. When you feel that you have mastered step 1, move away from the wall and use your elbows only to help you balance.
3. Cut back to one elbow.
4. Try putting on one sock without the wall; take a break and do the second sock.
5. Do both socks while standing in the middle of the room.
6. Repeat from step 1, adding putting on and then tying your shoes.
7. Stand on one leg for 10 seconds with your eyes open, then do the same on the other leg.
8. Repeat step 7 with your eyes closed.
9. Lift one foot off the ground, eyes closed, and hold for 10 seconds. Switch feet and hold for 10 seconds.
10. Build up to 30 seconds for each foot.
11. Repeat with arms out to the side, then with arms in prayer position. Work on holding this position for as long as you can.
12. For the full tree pose, bend one knee and place the sole of your foot on your straight leg, at or above the knee, hands in the prayer position. Use this position to balance yourself physically and mentally whenever you are feeling overwhelmed.

PART 3

*I*n this section I invite you to join the club. Not the fitness club or the golf and country club but the club whose members have their eyes on the future and know how to take special care of their health. We all know people who stay fit and slender throughout their entire lives, seemingly with little effort. Why shouldn't we all share their secrets?

As a reader of *Ace Your Health* you have your ears to the ground for the smart and simple things that will help you age gracefully, prevent cancer and heart disease, and stay healthy as long as possible. You are learning to make better choices by drawing on new and emerging information and on ancient wisdom. You are not afraid to go out into the sunshine (but smartly!) because you know that the sunshine is the best source of vitamin D and that vitamin D is a potent cancer fighter. You are not afraid to eat carbs but you eat the right ones in the right amounts. You avoid white sugar, pack your day with all of the potent foods that nature offers, and ramp up your game with the ideal amount of the best protein. You know how to make the most of every moment, movement, and mouthful and are happy to share what you know.

ACE OF CLUBS

TELOMERES AND TELOMERASE: Father time of the future

It is time to look into the future. Where is health going? What is the frontier? Here are two new words you should add to your vocabulary: telomeres and telomerase. The 2009 Nobel Prize for Medicine was awarded for the discovery of how telomeres and telomerase protect our long-term health – but you don't have to have a medical degree to grasp what they are about.

Grade-school biology taught us that all cells divide and replicate based on the information located within their unique DNA. What we now know is that the DNA strands are protected at their ends so they don't unravel. They are protected by telomeres just as a shoelace, made up of many thinner strands, is protected by those little plastic tips. Who hasn't tried to rethread a sneaker with a lace that has become frayed? It is virtually impossible, with both shoelaces and cell divisions, to get all the little threads to do what you want them to do, in a timely fashion, with 100 percent accuracy. Without telomeres, your cells could replicate into mutant cells and cause a whole host of problems, from allergies to cancer.

As we age, telomeres naturally become shorter and shorter and are at risk of fraying. Once they are no longer capable of passing along viable information, they take themselves out of the game. This is the leading theory of how the entire aging process works. There is a superhero enzyme called telomerase, which helps regenerate telomeres and is therefore key to keeping the information as viable as possible, as long as possible. Interestingly, some studies have pointed toward stress as one of the largest factors in out-of-whack telomere length and telomerase activity. This research is in its infancy, so we don't really know yet what its implications are, but the possibilities are exciting!

We all manage our stress differently and the Jack of Diamonds goes into that topic in more depth. For the purposes of protecting our telomeres, I will cover some of the stressors that are less typically considered.

PERCEIVED STRESS

It isn't the fact that stress exists but how we deal with it that matters. Time off, perspective, laughter, friendship, and even a glass of wine help us deal with stress. This may sound simplistic, but I believe that life really is simple and it is only we humans who complicate it. If anxiety plagues you, I urge you to get some professional help; stress can wreak havoc on your system in the long term. There is an ancient proverb that says, "He who worries suffers twice" – once in advance of the event and then again when the event does happen (sometimes as a *result* of all that worry!).

CHRONIC PAIN

We may not think of ongoing pain as stress but we all know how much shorter our fuse is when we have a headache or backache. If modern medicine hasn't helped, try a chiropractor, massage therapist, or acupuncturist – and keep trying. Whatever you can do to reduce your flare-ups, or your perception of your flare-ups, will reduce the stress that they cause on your body.

UNDERNOURISHMENT

Each and every cell in your body is working all the time to replicate itself and they need the right fuel to do a good job. This is the way we should be thinking of food; it's not just pleasure for our taste buds, it's fuel for every cell's engine. And if the fuel we're taking in is of low quality and filled with impurities, our machines won't run as well.

THE ANTIDOTE

High-nutrient, high-antioxidant, minimally processed foods are the fuel that cells need, so it follows that these nutrients are also the fuel of healthy telomeres, even if it hasn't been *proven* yet (it will be). I am not waiting for a double-blind, longitudinal study to tell me what my grandmother already knew, but it is nice to know that my daughter's generation will have that information to guide them. Until that time, a prudent approach tells us that we must give our bodies (and the telomeres within them) all that they need to protect themselves from degeneration and invasion. These nutrients are as old as the hills; they are in the colourful fruits and vegetables that Mother Nature has put there for us.

There is no upper limit on whole, fresh vegetables; you should eat them as much and as often as you can. Carte blanche. Free rein. They contain the telomere-protecting phytonutrients that scientists are discovering and studying one by one. Our grandmothers told us, "Eat your vegetables; they'll make your hair curl." Grandmothers of the future will say, "Eat your vegetables; they'll protect your telomeres."

WILTED WILD GREEN SALAD

This salad is filled with nutrients. All of these ingredients can be found growing wild across North America. Feel free to forage for greenery in local fields if you are sure they have not been sprayed with pesticides. If the fruit and veggie mart is more your style, the greens are widely available there too. There are many varieties of dandelion but all of them are deliciously bitter. Feel free to fiddle with the amounts of the different greens to suit your palate.

	Ingredients	*Benefits*
½ cup	chopped green onions (white and green parts)	vitamin K
3–4 cups	dandelion leaves	polyphenols; cleanse liver
2 cups	watercress and/or arugula	phytonutrients; protect telomeres
2 tbsp	grapeseed oil	polyunsaturated oil
3 tbsp	apple cider or sherry vinegar	aids digestion
1 tbsp	maple syrup	high-mineral sweetener
¼ tsp	sea salt	trace minerals
¼ tsp	black pepper	stimulates digestion

Rinse vegetables and allow to drain in colander. In a large frying pan with a lid, stir together dressing ingredients and warm over medium heat for 2 minutes. Chop green onions finely and dandelion leaves into thirds. Toss greens into dressing, turn down heat to low, cover and wilt for 2 minutes. Stir in watercress/arugula and serve immediately.

Preparation time: 4 minutes   Servings: 6

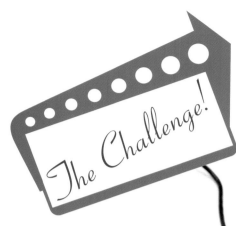

KEEP YOUR EYES OPEN for any and all news on telomeres. Occasionally google the phrase "news on telomere length" for new research that didn't even exist when this page was written. It is coming fast and furious now! But be skeptical of any supplements or drugs that promise to sustain youthful telomere length. That kind of innovation takes a long time to find, create, prove, and improve. I will have written another book by then.

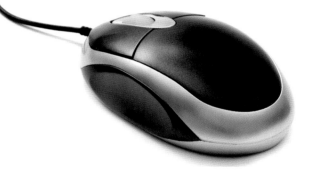

KING OF CLUBS

VITAMIN D: D' Whole Story

We all know that vitamin D comes from the sun but we also know that the sun is really, really bad for us, right? Wait a minute, maybe it isn't so clear-cut. Recent studies have implicated vitamin D deficiency in everything from cancer to multiple sclerosis. What gives?

It is hypothesized that the reason rates of cancer, dementia, osteoarthritis, and diabetes increase the farther away from the equator that a population lives is related to the relative intake of vitamin D. Other studies show that both cholesterol and blood pressure numbers are worse in the same patients over the winter. These facts make sense when you consider that the body needs vitamin D and other nutrients that come from the sun.

Nutritionists and doctors currently recommend vitamin D supplementation at 1,000 IU (international units) per day. Supplements come in drops (ideal for babies) as well as pills. Each of us has different needs and a simple blood test can tell you what your serum-25 hydroxy-vitamin D level is. Ask your doctor if you are at the cancer-protective levels (150-200 nmol/L). She'll think either that you are really smart or that you spend too much time on the Internet, but you will gain important information about your health.

But where is the fun in supplements? How about a more flavourful and fun approach?

STEP 1: *Practise unprotected sunshine*
It doesn't take a lot of time for the exposed skin of the arms and face to make 10,000 IU of vitamin D all by itself. And because your body is self-regulating, your skin will stop absorbing more when you have stored enough. A mere 15 minutes per day in summer is sufficient. If you live north of the 33rd parallel (north of, say, Atlanta or Los Angeles), you will need to increase that up to 30 or 45 minutes in the late spring and early fall. Unfortunately, winter above the 33rd parallel doesn't provide strong enough sunshine no matter how long you stay outside.

A supplement may be the best way to cover you off if a trip to the south isn't in the cards.

Needless to say, you don't want to spend an entire summer day at the beach in the sun without protection. But worn daily, that protection is preventing you from making vitamin D and limiting your immunity. The solution – to this and many other issues – is a 20-minute walk in the morning sun, without sunscreen. Play it smart: if you are just walking from your car to the mall or around the block with the dog, leave your legs exposed and protect your face only. Cover up during the height of the sun's rays but get some exposure at the beginning or at the end of each and every day.

Do not go directly from the sunshine to a soapy shower; wait a couple of hours. Converting vitamin D from sunshine requires fatty sweat. A cousin of cholesterol is excreted by the skin; it absorbs the sun, converts it, and is then reabsorbed as vitamin D by the skin – your own microscopic vitamin-making factory.

STEP 2: *Eat foods high in vitamin D*
Vitamin D resides only in a few of the good fatty foods and these may not be a part of your regular diet. Fish liver oils, fatty fishes like salmon, caviar,

and mushrooms are your go-to natural sources. There are all kinds of vitamin D-fortified foods, like milk and soy and rice milks, that are worth sourcing, too. Mushrooms are the only plant-based source and their vitamin D is not the highly absorbable sort, so if you're vegetarian or vegan, you're going to have to work a little harder (and perhaps fork over cash for that winter vacation in the sun!).

If you like sardines, you win on vitamin D and other counts because they are also high in CoQ10 (an enzyme that benefits your heart) and omega-3s (for your heart and everything else), and their small size means they haven't accumulated much mercury. A can or two per week is an affordable, tasty option. If you hate sardines, then salmon is another good source, as is cod liver oil, but that will be a hard sell.

STEP 3: *Take a vitamin D supplement*
If you are unwilling or unable to get enough sun or eat vitamin D-rich foods you will have to supplement. This is one pill that is worth every penny. One year's worth of adult vitamin D drops can be found in a small bottle costing about seven cents per day. Kids enjoy licking the drop off the back of their (clean) hands like a kitten, and adults are happy not to have to consume another pill.

TARAMASALATA

This traditional Greek dip is best made with fresh garlic, fresh lemon, and true extra virgin olive oil, but using garlic powder, bottled juice, and non–extra virgin olive oil is better than not making the dip at all. Starting with leftover mashed potatoes is quick, but if you don't have any on hand, simply bake a whole potato in the microwave and scoop out the pulp to cool before proceeding.

	Ingredients	*Benefits*
¼ cup	cod or carp roe	vitamin D; anticarcinogenic
1 cup	mashed potatoes	potassium for fluid balance
1	garlic clove, mashed	antibacterial
⅓ cup	extra virgin olive oil	glowing skin
½	lemon, juiced	alkalizes blood
½ tsp	honey	antibacterial
pinch	cayenne	stimulates salivary glands
pinch	oregano	boosts immunity

In a small food processor, mix roe with mashed potatoes and garlic. Blend in olive oil and lemon juice. Add honey and seasonings. Add water by the teaspoon if needed to thin.

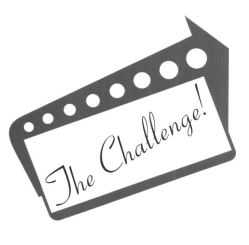

The Challenge!

THE CHALLENGE OF THE week is to look at your food sources of vitamin D. Estimate the number of IU you consume from measurable fortified sources (just read the label) and then add at least two servings from the list below per day. If you are falling short, think seriously about taking a supplement.

SOURCE	APPROXIMATE IU	AMOUNT
DAIRY		
FORTIFIED DAIRY ALTERNATIVES		
SARDINES		
OTHER FISH		
COD LIVER OIL		
TARAMASALATA		

QUEEN OF CLUBS

FIBRE: The royal flush

The benefits of a high-fibre diet are not only in the "prevention" category but also in the "solution" category. Eating lots of fibre can help **prevent** a raft of serious and debilitating diseases like diverticulitis, high cholesterol, many types of cancers (most notably colon), obesity, high blood pressure, and diabetes. And if you are diagnosed with any of these, a nutritionist will suggest a higher-fibre diet to help manage them. Some researchers have speculated that the increase in these diseases directly coincides with the decrease of fibre in our diet.

Fibre's job is to move foods through the digestive tract, meanwhile increasing the sense of fullness, or satiety, and scouring out cholesterol and other waste, thereby reducing blood sugar swings and overall inflammation. Recent studies have drawn a direct link between belly fat and fibre intake: when fibre goes down, belly fat goes up and vice versa. There is no downside to eating fibre.

When I mention fibre to most people they counter with, "Oh, I am fine, I eat (insert breakfast cereal here)," which, depending upon the brand, can get you almost *halfway* to your daily intake. We need a daily minimum of 25 grams of fibre, though some say 35 to 40 grams is a better goal. However, Canadians are averaging only between 4.5 and 11 grams per day. You can't stop thinking about fibre just because you have a few flakes in your cereal bowl.

There are two kinds of fibre, soluble and insoluble, but don't waste time counting a nd sorting how much of each that you get: if you are getting one, you are likely getting the other. You need both because they do different things.

SOLUBLE FIBRE dissolves, so it can be broken down by our digestive enzymes. It is in things like fruit, oats, beans, sweet potatoes, chia, and psyllium. Soluble fibre helps fight heart disease because its jelly-like consistency allows it to capture cholesterol on its way through our blood system.

INSOLUBLE FIBRE cannot be broken down in our bodies, so it is the one that bulks up the bowel and moves waste through. It is found in whole grains (like bran), nuts and seeds, wheat, corn, and the skins of some vegetables (like tomatoes) and the strings in celery.

To make friends with fibre:

- Keep your high-fibre cereal but I want you to use it a little differently. As the Ace of Spades explained, cereal for breakfast does not offer enough protein to start the day. Find a high-fibre cereal that tastes good and have it instead as a snack throughout the day. A handful can go a long way toward filling your gut, which turns off the "feed me!" signal coming from the belly.

- Bring a little chia into your day. These seeds contain both kinds of fibre and one tablespoon delivers four grams, which is a whopping amount. If you find bran fibre harsh or explosive, chia is your solution.

- If you haven't already switched to whole grains, what are you waiting for? There are lots of whole-grain products on the shelves. Go half and half for a while to smooth the transition; a sandwich with one white slice and one dark slice of bread looks beautiful and tastes great! A handful of whole-grain pasta can go into the pot first and be cooked for a minute or two extra and then you can add the white stuff. (Some of the new white pastas on the market are made with a fibre called inulin, which may or may not have the benefits of the whole-food sources; the jury is still out.)
- Increasing all fruits and vegetables is happening on each and every page of *Ace Your Health,* so you can leave that one to me.

BEST POPCORN EVER!

The lining in a microwave popcorn bag contains a Teflon-like substance that has been linked to cancer. Plus, the fats and salt (even if the package says low-fat or low-salt) are way too high. When you see how easy and delicious it is to make a guilt-free, low-sodium, low-fat, highly nourishing popcorn containing three grams of fibre, you will never look back. Kids under three should not have popcorn or peanuts until you are sure that they can fully chew and not choke and are cleared for allergies.

Ingredients		*Benefits*
¼ cup	popcorn	low-cal, high-fibre
1 tbsp	extra virgin olive oil	best raw fat
1 tbsp	nutritional yeast	B vitamins; add salty/cheesy taste
½ tsp	Sea(soning) Mix	multi-mineral salt
¼ cup	unsalted peanuts	protein to balance carbs

Place popcorn in a brown paper bag and twist the opening closed. Microwave on high for 2–3 minutes until you hear the pops slow down. Empty into a bowl and discard any unpopped kernels. Drizzle with olive oil and sprinkle with Sea(soning)Mix and nutritional yeast. Stir in peanuts and sneak a bagful into a movie!

Preparation time: **2 minutes** Servings: 2

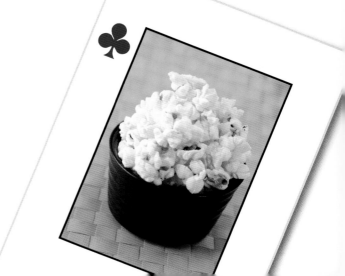

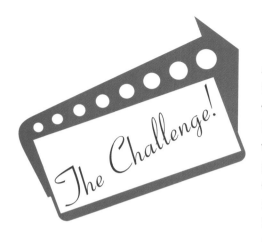

AS UNSAVOURY AS IT may sound (and as embarrassing as it is to my teenage daughter), I am fascinated by poop. You can tell a lot about what went into a body by what comes out. The goal is to obtain at least one good bowel movement each day that comes unbidden by your morning coffee. Those who think they are "regular" because they go immediately after a cup of joe are going to have to reassess. The poop I am looking for comes without a stomach cramp, it is whole and somewhat solid and much fatter than you would think (the bowel learns to stretch to accommodate the fibre and that's healthy, muscle-building, colon-cleaning action). It is smooth, sinks, and is not very smelly. Its colour is somewhere between caramel and tan and it is six to eight inches long.

If you are getting that sneaking suspicion that I am going to make you look in the bowl, you are exactly right! This week, instead of counting all the grams on packages, let's see the results. Record for the next week (or two or three, because it can take a while to get the magic we are looking for) when, how, and how much of a "royal flush" you are able to obtain.

	WHEN	FREQUENCY	VOLUME
MONDAY			
TUESDAY			
WEDNESDAY			
THURSDAY			
FRIDAY			
SATURDAY			
SUNDAY			

JACK OF CLUBS

SUPERFRUITS: Nature's little superheroes

I have to admit, I am not a big fruit eater but, in my defence, I make up for it in vegetables, which is a lower-calorie, lower-sugar solution to getting the same nutrients. Mostly, it is because I live in a northern climate and I can't bear to eat an out-of-season peach from California when the real thing is grown an hour away in August. I go through barrels of peaches then but, come September, they are banished. And blueberries?

We pick them wild off the land in my husband's east coast hometown or purchase baskets when we drop our daughter off up north at her summer camp. No imported winter fruit that has travelled thousands of miles can even come close to the sensory experience of summer bounty, so I don't bother trying. However, I do know that there are benefits of these foods, so I have found creative ways to work them into my life without compromise.

Fruits come in such gorgeous hues to attract animals *and* fight off pests. It is these smart, colour-coded molecules that we want to eat and the more the better, provided that they are in their whole, natural form. These pigments are health-protecting, life-giving cells but they are as delicate as they are strong. It isn't just vitamin C and its brethren that we are looking for; it is also the phytonutrients, polyphenols, minerals, and fibre. There is heated debate about whether isolating one nutrient in a supplement is as good for you as the whole food, and I weigh in on the side of food every time as long as you can get enough of it (see Ace of Diamonds). I can't find one single thing that nature has created that was actually *improved* by man. Isolating one nutrient means *processing* it. To my logic, the less affected a fruit is by heat, light, travel, pesticides, and processing, the better it will be for you.

My favourite ways to get the best out of fruit, even in Canada in January, are these:

FROZEN BERRIES. Store-bought packages contain berries that are usually picked at the height of ripeness and quickly frozen to preserve as much flavour and nutrition as possible. If you can find your own in the wild (or at a roadside stand), that's the best option. Freezing them on cookie sheets and then moving them to freezer baggies can mean cheap, easy access to the best and the brightest right through to next year. Adding them to smoothies and yogurt doesn't diminish their value and they thaw extremely quickly.

NEW AND SEXY FRUITS. Acai berries and goji berries *are* what they are cracked up to be as long as they are in their whole, unpowdered, unheated glory. While they won't cure your cancer or your cold sore all by themselves overnight, they are worth adding for their powerful health effects. Unfortunately, acai berries are never available fresh or frozen in my grocery or health store. They are always powdered, juiced, or otherwise manipulated, and I have no way of knowing how they were handled. So I prefer goji berries, which are available dried and whole in the bulk store, health food store, and often in the Asian section of the grocery store. The Chinese use them to sweeten and balance otherwise salty dishes. They are high in fibre, antioxidants, vitamins, and minerals, and worth adding to stir fries and salads.

Juices are usually not the best way to get your fruit, with a few exceptions. Knowing that nutrients' enemies are heat, light, air, and time means choosing your juice wisely. Many manufacturers simply take the fruit that is unsellable for eating fresh and process it using heat-pasteurizing that kills bacteria, but can also kill nutrients. Often the juices are stored for long periods. The vitamin C is added before bottling, which looks good on the label.

If you are using juices to obtain phytonutrients, it is worth looking for an expanded nutrition panel on the packaging showing superior nutrient scores (fibre is a good one to look for) and concern for freshness. These juices will always be sold from the refrigerated section.

The top fruits to eat fresh are those that contain a high amount of water, nutrients, and fibre in relation to their calories. So bananas, for instance, while great potassium providers, have more carbohydrate and sugar and less fibre for the number and kind of nutrients they provide. None of these fruits are *bad* for you, but blackberries are the *best* choice: low in calories, carbs, and sugar yet high in fibre and phytonutrients.

Fresh, whole fruit is the true winner, but what about dried fruits? They are concentrated sources of nutrients but they can also contain drying and processing chemicals, as well as mould spores. If you have an allergy to mould or have frequent yeast infections, beware of dried fruit. The concentrated sugars will feed the yeast, and the naturally occurring mould has an opportunity to grow within this environment. If you are a dried fruit lover, the best way to consume it is in small amounts (like three figs or dates) before a workout. The immediately useable energy will give you a boost with calories that can be burned off in the first hour of exercise, along with minerals that will help you recover faster. It is best to avoid the sugar-spiking fruit chews that only stick in your teeth and buy your dentist a boat to go with the cottage you paid for last year.

FRUIT	BANANA (1 MED)	BLACKBERRIES (1 CUP)	BLUEBERRIES (1 CUP)
CALORIES	90	62	83
CARBOHYDRATES (g)	23	14	21
FIBRE (g)	2.6	7.6	3.5
SUGAR (g)	12.4	7	14.4
PHYTONUTRIENTS	medium	high	high

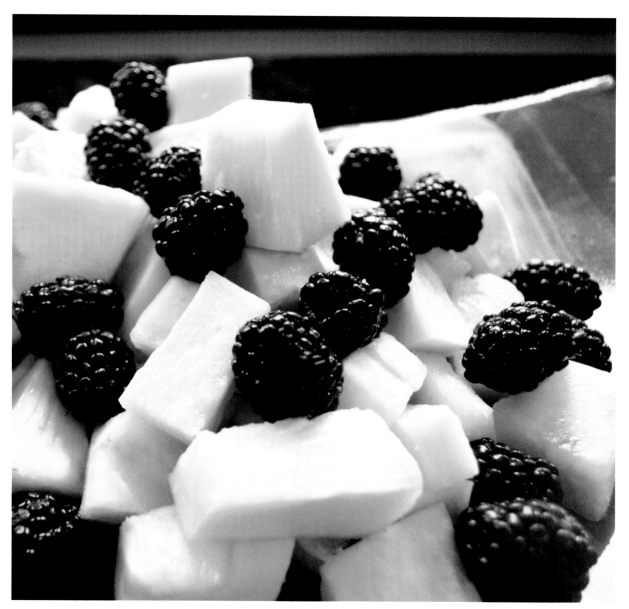

BLUEBERRY DREAM

This is a turbo-powered, nutrient-dense dish that looks like a high-end dessert, candy crackle and all! Make it with pomegranate or blueberry juice

Ingredients

		Benefits
1 cup	pure, unsweetened blueberry or pomegranate juice	high in antioxidants
¼ cup	pure maple syrup	trace minerals
2 cups	plain yogurt	probiotic; for intestinal health
1 cup	blueberries, fresh or frozen	low-cal, high-fibre pure nutrient

To make candy crackle: Measure ¼ cup of blueberry or pomegranate juice into a small pot and stir in maple syrup. Bring to a boil and simmer for about 10 minutes (until the hard-crack stage or mixture becomes very foamy and has large bubbles).While the mixture is simmering, pour remaining juice into yogurt and stir in blueberries. Divide into 4 martini glasses and store in fridge until ready to serve.

When syrup-juice mixture is ready, carefully pour onto a baking sheet lined with parchment or onto a flexible silicon sheet. Let harden for 10–15 minutes, then fold paper or sheet over and smash crackle into small pieces. Top yogurt mixture with crackle and serve.

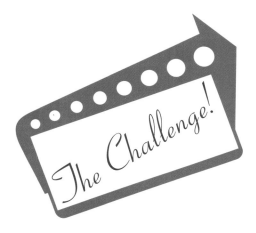

The Challenge!

GO TO YOUR FRIDGE right now and pull out all the fruit. If there is none, make a trip to the store and pick up fruits of at least three different colours. Peel and chop if necessary, then put the fruit into a bowl and pour some lemon juice over it to prevent browning. Serve this fruit salad as a dessert. If you get into the habit of having fruit at the ready, it is more likely to get eaten. It's doing nobody any good down there in the crisper. Dress the fruit salad up with a bit of fat-free vanilla yogurt and a dash of cinnamon and nutmeg. Serve from martini glasses and it will feel like a treat!

TEN OF CLUBS

————

The first thing that people ask me when they find out what I do for a living is "Which diet should I be on?" Who could blame them? We have been through decades of directives from low-fat to low-carb to nonsense. My answer to their question is always "The only diet you should be on is your own." In other words, I can't answer that question while I am drinking wine at a party and eyeing the cheese platter. I would have to look at your whole day within the scope of your whole life including your own goals. In the end, a series of small changes will guide each person's very own "diet."

That said, when I take a look at what we are eating as a population, most Canadians rely very heavily on carbohydrates (and, shockingly, the white ones). We have our high-fibre cereal in the morning, a double (and often quadruple dose of) bread in a sandwich at lunch, and too much of the not-so-great white carbs at dinner. Some whole-grain bread is good for you and delicious, too, but we tend to eat *too much* of the *wrong* sort of whole grains. The trick with carbs is to choose the best whole-grain source and have no more than two to two and a half cups per day. If you stop relying upon bread, and using it to fill you up, you may be better able to control your blood sugar levels and your weight. Plus, you will discover your true hunger

and how to manage it, without feeling bloated and stuffed. Then, and only then, should you add bread back into your diet and truly enjoy it.

Don't confuse this approach with removing all carbohydrates. Our bodies prefer carbohydrates because they are the most efficient energy source. Plus, we get much more from whole grains and fruits than just calories, so throwing these babies out with the bathwater is not the way to go. There are some amazing yet seldom eaten starchy side dishes that make awesome additions to any meal. Whole grain rice now comes in all sorts of shapes, sizes, and colours and is extremely easy to simmer in a rice cooker, where it is ready for you at the end of a day. A quick toss of veggies in a pan and a meal is on the table in minutes.

Other whole grains include these:

QUINOA (pronounced *keen-wa*) originates from the Andes Mountains of South America. It is gluten-free, easily digested, and a great substitute for couscous (which is really just tiny white pasta in a granulated form). Quinoa is the highest-protein grain and has a nearly ideal amino acid balance (more like a seed than a grain). It is also a good source of fibre, calcium, phosphorus, iron, and vitamins B and E.

Directions for 3–4 servings:

1 cup quinoa + 2 cups water or low-sodium chicken broth

Rinse quinoa thoroughly in pot and pour off as much water as possible, through a sieve. Add water or stock to pot and bring to a boil. Cover and simmer for 8 minutes. Stir in seasonings as you wish. Try garlic and oregano, 1 tablespoon of yogurt, ½ teaspoon extra virgin olive oil.

MILLET One of the least allergenic and easily digestible grains, millet is also gluten-free. It is high in B vitamins and has a good amino acid profile. Great in place of rice in casseroles, soups, and stuffings.

Directions for 3–4 servings:
3½ cups water + 1 cup millet

Bring water to a boil and stir in millet. Simmer, uncovered, for 25–30 minutes. To use as a stuffing side dish: Brown 1 chopped onion, 2 stalks celery, and 1 grated carrot in a skillet with 1 tablespoon butter. Stir in poultry seasoning and ½ teaspoon herbal sea salt. Stir millet into veggies and serve in a casserole dish.

BARLEY Barley is a very high-fibre, high-magnesium grain. It becomes slightly creamy when cooked, and lends itself to a risotto-like side dish.

Directions for 5–6 servings:

1 cup pot barley + 3 cups chicken stock + ¼ cup grated Parmesan cheese + 1 tbsp nutritional yeast

Simmer barley in chicken stock for about 50 minutes or until soft, adding water if necessary. Drain if any liquid is left over. Remove from heat. Let cool 4–6 minutes. Add Parmesan cheese, yeast, and stir. Excellent with grilled shrimp and green onions.

BABY BOK CHOY WITH BAKED TOFU

Prepare this easy-to-assemble, low-cal, nutrient-dense, stir-fry-like meal
at a moment's notice. Serve it over any one of the "good grains" above and rotate it
in to your repertoire weekly—your body and taste buds will thank you.
If you have a moment to toast the sesame seeds, it will enhance the flavour.

	Ingredients	*Benefits*
14 oz	firm tofu	protects against breast cancer
4 tbsp	low-sodium soy sauce,	
	or liquid amino acids	trace protein
1 tbsp	honey	antimicrobial
1 tsp	garlic powder	boosts immunity
10	large stalks baby bok choy	low-cal; high in vitamin A
1 tbsp	sesame oil	lignans; control blood pressure
1 tbsp	sesame seeds	protect liver against oxidative damage

Wrap tofu in paper towel and place on plate to dry for 10 minutes at room temperature. Slice tofu into 1-inch squares, ¼ inch thick. Mix soy sauce, honey and garlic powder together in a small bowl and add tofu to marinate for 10 minutes at room temperature. Rinse baby bok choy leaves very well. Heat oven to 425°F. Place bok choy onto cookie sheet and arrange marinated tofu pieces on top. Bake 15 minutes, uncovered. Drizzle with sesame oil and top with sesame seeds after you remove from oven.

Preparation time: **20 minutes** Servings: **4**

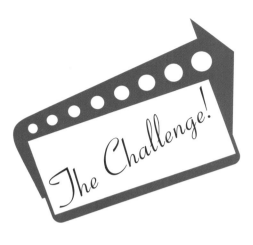

MEASURE YOUR CARBOHYDRATE DAY in handfuls. If you were to put your piece of bread or bowl of pasta or cereal in one hand, how many times would you fill it up each day? A handful is about one-half cup to three-quarters of a cup.

This week, banish all white carbs and stick to a whole-grain regime. (Bonus points if you stick to it from this day forward!) A guideline for an appropriate amount of carbs for the average, moderately active woman would be four handfuls per day if trying to lose weight, and up to five or six when she reaches her goal weight. Men can eat five to six handfuls during a weight-loss regime, depending upon their size and activity level, and go up to seven or eight to maintain. Everyone's body is different and you need to watch your scale and your hunger level to know how you are doing.

	TOTAL HANDFULS	TYPE OF CARB	ADD 2 POINTS FOR EACH WHITE CARB
MONDAY			
TUESDAY			
WEDNESDAY			
THURSDAY			
FRIDAY			
SATURDAY			
SUNDAY			

Scoring

	Women	*Men*
A+:	below 28	below 35
B:	below 35	below 42
C:	below 42	below 49
D:	above 50	below 56

NINE OF CLUBS

PROTECTING YOUR BONES AND JOINTS: Mobility matters

It's when you catch yourself groaning as you rise from your seat or moaning as you bend to get the towel off the floor that your realize you *sound* older than you look or feel. The creakiness creeps in and we tend to accept it in stages, so it doesn't freak us out until we are too tired or too much in pain to do anything about it. (The trick is to reach that marker when you are 96, not 36!)

There are four things you can do to make a huge impact on your bones and joints and they are worked in throughout *Ace Your Health*, but this card is intended to help you focus on the key points in protecting movement: managing your weight, reducing inflammation, increasing lubrication, and being active.

MANAGE YOUR WEIGHT

In order to ace your health, you don't necessarily need to lose weight. There are lots of technically "overweight" but very fit people who do just fine carrying around a bit extra for a rainy day. Weight loss comes as a matter of course when you do the right things for other and better reasons. So, if you have played the game well, you have probably already dropped a few pounds and not felt deprived. Even losing 10 percent of

your body weight is enough to make a huge difference in your health markers of blood pressure, cholesterol counts, and triglycerides, and it will also make a difference on your joints.

Our bodies are made to carry around a reasonable amount of weight, and your heart, muscles, blood vessels, and joints are designed to support that number. Added stress by way of added weight only accelerates the wear and tear on everything. Think of it no differently from your car's shock system. A heavy truck has a shock system that is made to handle heavy loads, but if you are constantly throwing cement blocks, heavy tools, and four huge people into mommy's little hatchback, those shocks are going to give out. No amount of oil is going to help; that baby is going to sit low to the ground and groan over every bump in the road. The best thing you can do if your weight is holding you back is to review all of the cards so far and take them seriously. Implement every challenge and drop just 10 percent of the weight in your own little hatchback. This will give you the impetus to tackle the next step of protecting your mobility.

REDUCE INFLAMMATION

So many of our modern diseases, from arthritis to lupus and right on up to heart disease and dementia, arise from inflammation. Inflammation is the body's way of dealing with whatever isn't right. A fever is trying to tackle the germs of an infection, a cut on your finger gets hot and red as your personal little firefighters rush in to staunch the flow, and swollen joints are the body's attempt at bringing lubrication to the place of pain. Our bodies can't keep up with the inflammation caused by what the average North American eats, drinks, and inhales. In other sections of *Ace Your Health* I have recommended anti-inflammatory foods like green tea, fish, and chia seeds, and discouraged the consumption of "white foods." All of these changes are helping you to keep inflammation in check.

There are a few specific foods that people who suffer from an inflammatory disease may want to consider. Taking a page out of the naturopathic approach to joint pain may mean excluding the vegetables in the group called the nightshade family (tomatoes, potatoes, eggplant, and peppers), especially during flare-ups. While healthy and delicious, they are considered to be inflammatory and it is worth a two-week experiment to see if eliminating them helps you. Sweet potatoes don't seem to have the same effect and are a good substitute. There's nothing as delicious or healthy as tomatoes, but once you know that they are a trigger for you, eat them wisely rather than daily.

The foods to be sure to add are cherries, celery, celery seeds, and fresh ginger. Getting a serving or two of any combination of these every day can't hurt and may help reduce inflammation immensely.

INCREASE LUBRICATION

I am always baffled by the array of creams and potions that are slathered on our exteriors when, if we spent that money on what goes inside us, we'd net better results while spending less and enjoying delicious food. The juice our bodies need comes from the good fat found in eggs, fish, nuts, and seeds, as well as chia. Adding more of these and less of the processed foods is a simple way to stop the creak. A lifetime of enjoying these foods is our best bet for preventing joint deterioration.

GET ACTIVE

"Use it or lose it" applies to just about everything in life but is never more true than with exercise. Bones and the fluid in joints are enhanced and regenerated with every movement, for our entire lifespan. As prevention, exercise – and attention to posture – are important. We spend an inordinate amount of time at our desks reusing small joints in awkward positions and then wondering why we have headaches or why our shoulders are so stiff that lifting a bag of groceries out of the trunk requires Herculean effort. We have to move a lot more during each day and shake off, shrug off, stretch out as often as possible. You should aim to have a good supportive chair, positioned at the right height, and have your wrists supported while you type, which will help in preventing the cramps, aches, and pains that result. Tucking your chin toward your chest 20 or 30 times an hour can relieve the neck stress before shoulders get sore, and it's these small and simple changes that can make a huge difference.

CHERRY SMOOTHIE

A smoothie makes for a great start to your day or a refreshing afternoon snack.
Wouldn't it be wonderful to have one of these instead of a cup of coffee at 3 p.m.?
Pure, anti-inflammatory fuel to get you through to the end of your slog.

Ingredients

		Benefits
1 cup	sour cherries in juice	anti-inflammatory
1 cup	pomegranate juice	high in antioxidants
1	banana	high-potassium sweetener/thickener
½ cup	hemp protein powder	gamma-linolenic acid; reduces inflammation
3 cups	pineapple juice	anti-inflammatory
¼ tsp	ground cloves	anti-inflammatory
¼ tsp	ground ginger	anti-inflammatory

Place cherries and pomegranate juice in blender and blend. Add banana and blend.
Add remaining ingredients and blend.

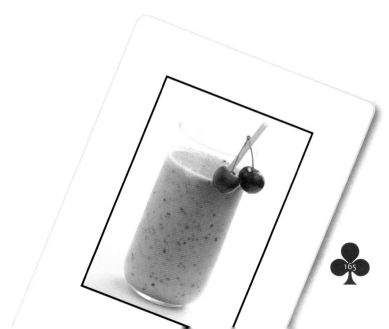

Preparation time: 2 minutes Servings: 4 to 6

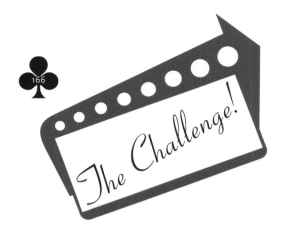

The Challenge!

MY OFFICE CHAIR IS called a Sguig, made by Keilhauer, and it is the best investment I have made in my health. It encourages "active sitting" and deters hunching. I use a wrist pad for my mouse and a footstool to raise my feet off the ground. Doing this helps me to write for hours at a time without suffering the consequences. My seat is set so that my computer screen is at a 45-degree angle to my eyes. It is the perfect setup for me and has prevented some of the cramping, headache, and general stiffness that come with sedentary work. The rest of my life is spent standing over hot pots or crouching with a camera at odd angles, but I deal with these with massages and by doing strength training at the gym.

Let's take a look at your seating arrangement:

- Do you sit all day at work?
- Is your chair a desk chair or a bus seat?
- Does your chair fully and adequately support you?
- Can you bring in a back support for your lower back? Even a rolled-up towel will do.
- Do you need something to raise your feet off the ground? If you are under five feet four inches like me, chances are that you do, because desks and chairs just aren't designed for shorter heights.
- Do you do a repetitive task all day? Can you take regular breaks to stretch the muscles in the opposite direction? Two minutes every hour is a good guideline.
- Do you have a support for your wrist or elbow where needed? These pads are practically free at the dollar store and can make a huge difference. Simply shifting the angle of your repeated actions for an hour or so per day can take the pressure off.
- What about "at rest" while you are watching TV? Do you slump or slouch? Could you lie on the ground and gently stretch you full body for even a few minutes?

List some things that you could do within your budget to help your body be active:

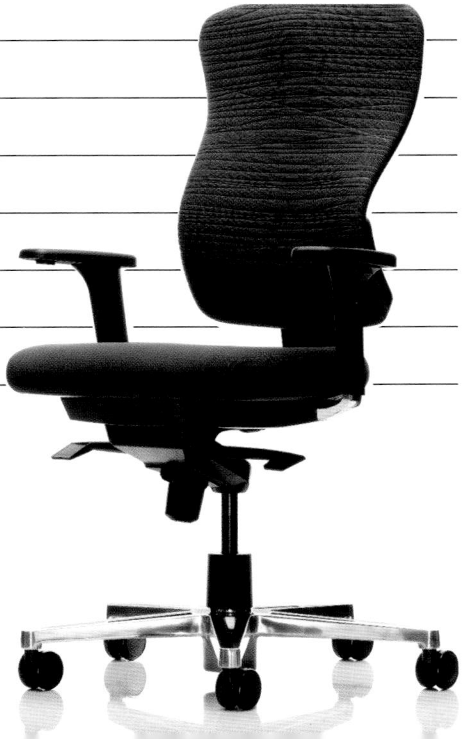

_____

_____

_____

_____

_____

_____

_____

_____

_____

_____

_____

EIGHT OF CLUBS

SUGAR AND SWEETENERS: The sweet things in life

You have heard the bad news about how many teaspoons of sugar there are in your breakfast cereal (before it even goes into your bowl), and how damaging the high-fructose corn syrup in your can of soda is, but let's take a closer look at sugar and what it does to our bodies.

Our bodies are not meant to process the intense sweetness of processed sugar; they are made to pull out the natural sugars that come along with other nutrients like the minerals in fruit, the fibre in flour. If we remove the minerals and fibre, the pancreas goes into overdrive and chugs out more insulin than the body knows what to do with. Do this too often and the pancreas just wears out, kind of like leaving a year's worth of receipts in a shoebox and then trying to do your books and your taxes in one day.

My clients are stunned by how much energy they find when they remove processed sugar from their diets. Having lived on the highs and lows of this drug for days or decades nets the same result: you end up needing more and more of it to get the same amount of "energy." I am not saying that you can't eat your own birthday cake or drink a sweetened beverage now and then, but you do

need to make sugar consumption the exception, not the rule. And you do need to mitigate the impact wisely.

White sugar can be replaced with one of the following ingredients in everything from your baking to your teacup. It is important to note that they all contain about the same amount of calories, about 16 to 20 per teaspoon, but, as usual, it is all about what comes *with* those calories.

EVAPORATED CANE SUGAR

This is essentially the same thing as granulated white sugar. Evaporated cane sugar comes from the same plant but rather than being bleached and depleted in the processing, the entire cane plant is pressed and the water evaporated. Cane sugar still has its minerals and trace amounts of fibre, so it has a few tools to help your body process the calories. Health food stores and bulk stores are good places to find it but Asian and

Indian markets are even better. In Indian shops, look for jaggery powder. It has an almost butterscotch taste with a molasses-like colour and smell and is incredible in a cup of coffee.

AGAVE NECTAR

This is the sweet and honey-like liquid from the agave cactus. Agave can be costly but it is the only sweetener I suggest for diabetics because it has been tested as having a low glycemic response, which means that it doesn't spike blood sugars as white granulated sugar does. I am not a fan of artificial sweeteners, mostly because they all have an acidic aftertaste. In large enough doses (estimated at more than 8 or 10 diet sodas per day), artificial sweeteners have been shown to be unsafe. Also, there is burgeoning evidence that the sensation of sweetness without the delivery of calories has a negative impact on our perception of caloric intake. In other words, it tastes sweet but your body doesn't get the calories it expects, which makes you want sugar even more. I would rather see you eat real, low-glycemic sweeteners and account for them in your daily intake.

PURE MAPLE SYRUP

My personal favourite, as I grew up having family in rural Quebec. Amber maple syrup is a concentrated flavour that adds to any pancake or coffee cup a certain *je ne sais quoi*. Real maple syrup brings with it excellent trace minerals that help you digest its carbohydrates and add to your nutritional bottom line. In particular, zinc, magnesium, and manganese are hard to get from plant sources, since many vegetables are grown in shallow, depleted soil. Maple trees get their nutrients from a rich, deep layer of bedrock *and* topsoil. Tapping the trunks before those minerals got to the leaves originated with the First Nations. Evaporating the sap concentrates these minerals in the syrup. Commercial "maple-flavoured" table syrups are usually made with artificially flavoured corn syrup, which is no better than pouring a can of soda pop on your pancakes.

HONEY

Nectar of the gods, honey has recently been discovered to have antibacterial agents that are as potent as penicillin, and it is under study as a way to fight "superbugs": micro-organisms that are resistant to antibiotics. But I wouldn't go spreading honey on scraped knees just yet. While there is much more to be learned about which strains of honey are the most effective, we do know that it contains something that does more than just taste great. Honey, like the other suggested sweeteners, also has minerals that we sorely need. Its active enzymes are delicate, so choose one that is as minimally processed as possible – not pasteurized, creamed, or otherwise heated – to get its full benefits.

SPICED NUTS

I always serve some version of spiced nuts as an appetizer before a dinner party. They are high enough in good fats to keep raging hunger at bay while helping the liver to process some of the alcohol inevitably served at cocktail hour. My guests usually eat only a tablespoon or so because they are so flavourful, and then they don't come to the table so full that they can't enjoy the fruits of my hard work. Also, the spices in the mix get the stomach juices ready and this homemade version is much lower in sodium than a store-bought mix.

Ingredients		*Benefits*
2 tbsp	butter	small amount extends other flavours
4 tbsp	maple syrup	zinc for insulin metabolism
2 tsp	curry powder	aids digestion
½ tsp	cayenne pepper	boosts metabolism
2 cups	chopped walnuts	slows metabolization of alcohol
½ tsp	sea salt	trace minerals

Melt butter in a large stainless steel pan and swirl in maple syrup. Allow to simmer for 2–3 minutes until mixture looks a little sticky and has thickened slightly. Turn off heat and swirl in spices, then add walnuts. Stir well with a heatproof spatula and turn out onto a cookie sheet or parchment paper to cool. Sprinkle with sea salt.

Preparation time: **3 minutes**   Servings: **12**

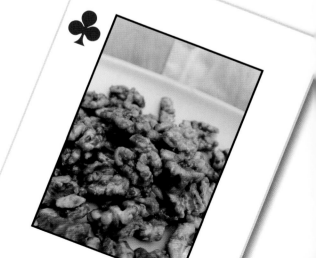

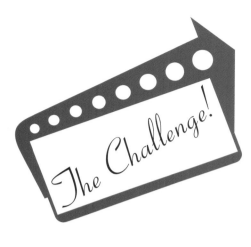

The Challenge!

OPTION A:
Eliminating the sugar consumed in beverages (and therefore as useless calories) would change the face of obesity and diabetes on this continent. It's a good place to start. If you are a coffee or tea drinker, keep track of how many teaspoonsful of sugar you use this week.

_____cups X _____ tsp X _____ days = _____ tsp

Look at all the lost opportunities to consume minerals with that sugar! If you are shocked at the amount of sugar you consume in hot beverages, try to reduce it by one teaspoon per day. Shoot for the lowest number you can. Next week, replace this amount with one of the better sources listed above.

OPTION B:
If you are not a coffee or tea drinker, find out how many teaspoons of sugar you are drinking each day from other liquids (juice, pop, etc.). These can really add up and are completely empty calories. Labels usually express sugar in grams and there are just over four grams of sugar in one teaspoon.

OPTION C:
If you have already removed drinkable sugars from your life, switch to one of the four suggested sweeteners for baking and brunching.

THE FINAL FRONTIER:
The next step is to hunt down all of the hidden sugars in your favourite foods.

SEVEN OF CLUBS

PROTEIN: Play your protein according to Hoyle

One of the more baffling debates in the fitness world is the role of protein in our diets. How much is enough? What's the best source? Is there such a thing as too much? Luckily, there are many ways to play your perfect protein day with a few simple rules.

For your cells to repair and replace themselves, you need at least .4 grams of protein per pound of your body weight daily. (Multiply your weight in pounds by 4 and divide by 10.) The maximum seems to be about two grams per pound. Any more than that and your kidneys can't process the waste; protein is not a clean-burning fuel.

You can get protein from many, many sources, not just meat, so mothers of teenaged vegetarians shouldn't worry. Proteins are made from a chain of amino acids, and animal-based sources have all of the links so they are the *easiest* ones to have in your hand but not the only ones. As you now know, it is really about what comes *with* that protein, and with animal sources, you always get cholesterol (even with chicken and fish) and sometimes more saturated fat than you want. Animal sources can also come with a lot of calories, something to consider if you are trying to lose weight.

Our bodies are able to combine the amino acids from plant-based sources to make a useable form of complete protein. I aim to include more plant-based sources of protein in my diet because they come without the cholesterol and are easier on the planet. It is necessary to shake it up a bit rather than rely on one source, to ensure that all essential amino acids are covered. Some examples are hemp seeds, soybeans, beans, nuts/seeds, in combination with the good grains. There is fat in nuts and they can be high in calories, but their every ounce of fat is anti-inflammatory, good fat that will help you clear out your cholesterol. That said, one small handful per day is plenty.

If you choose to include animal protein, lean sources are best to help you minimize the downside while maximizing the benefits. In order of lowest-calorie, lowest-saturated fat to highest, they are egg whites, whole eggs, fish, low-fat dairy, skinless chicken, pork tenderloin, beef tenderloin, and lamb loin. Reducing your reliance on animal sources of protein is a great way to save money, save the planet, and improve your health. But simply cutting out meat is not necessarily the right way to go! A steady diet of white rice and kidney beans will be deficient in one amino acid or another, which isn't a huge problem over a week in Mexico but may be over a lifetime. I have seen just as many overweight, undernourished vegetarians as meat eaters. And having too much protein from any one source won't do you any good either.

The key with protein, no matter the source, is to spread it out over the day; a little bit of protein at each meal is better for you than a whole bunch at suppertime. Protein is processed slowly by your digestive tract, so it helps control your blood sugar level. While processed and powdered protein isolates may be appropriate for those training for an Ironman challenge, they aren't the best sources for the rest of us. So much more comes from food in its whole, unprocessed, undried, unadulterated form that consuming concentrated sources of protein is not necessary. Use them only when you are in a real crunch and adding them to a breakfast smoothie is the only way to get protein in the morning. Don't be tricked into thinking that you *need* to use these powders to get the most out of your average workout. A simple glass of milk or soy milk and a handful of nuts will replenish what you lost in your biweekly spinning class.

PAN-FRIED TURMERIC FISH

I try to check the watch list at *www.montereybayaquarium.org* (click on "seafood watch") occasionally to avoid eating fish that are caught with practices that are damaging to fish stocks or to the health of our oceans. U.S. farm–raised catfish is safe, clean, ecologically sound, and deliciously unlike the oily counterpart bottom dweller we are accustomed to, so it has become a fave. Other white fishes may be substituted according to taste. This dish is delicious with dandelion greens from the Ace of Clubs.

Ingredients		*Benefits*
1	egg	complete protein
2 tbsp	turmeric (or curry powder)	anticarcinogenic
2 tbsp	whole-wheat flour	high-fibre coating for fish
¼ tsp	sea salt	contains potassium
¼ tsp	white pepper	stimulates salivary glands
1 lb	catfish fillets	complete protein
1 tbsp	butter	trace proteins
1 tbsp	grapeseed oil	polyunsaturated fat

Beat egg in a shallow bowl with 1 tbsp of water. Mix together turmeric, whole-wheat flour, sea salt, and white pepper in a separate bowl. Dredge fish in egg and then set into turmeric/flour mixture, turning to coat. Warm a large skillet over medium-high heat and add butter and oil. Quickly add the coated fish. Cook for 2–3 minutes and turn once to cook through for 2–3 more minutes. Set fish onto paper towel to absorb any excess fat.

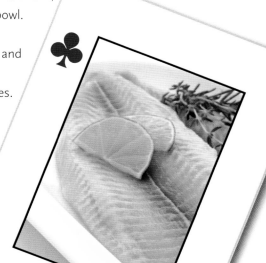

Preparation time: 12 minutes Servings: 4

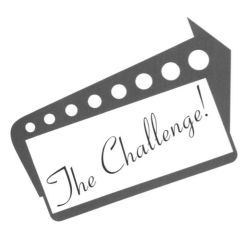

The Challenge!

WHAT KIND OF PROTEIN day did you have yesterday? Use the chart below and information on the nutrition panel of any packaged foods you ate to determine your protein score for the day. Then take a moment to plan tomorrow to be sure that you hit your target!

	YESTERDAY	ITEM	PROTEIN IN GRAMS (APPROX.)
BREAKFAST			
SNACK			
LUNCH			
SNACK			
SUPPER			

	TOMORROW	ITEM	PROTEIN IN GRAMS (APPROX.)
BREAKFAST			
SNACK			
LUNCH			
SNACK			
SUPPER			

SIX OF CLUBS

EGGS: The protein source of champions

Eggs were designed to support life; they contain everything needed to bring a being into existence. It follows, then, that they rank high on the list of good foods with nutritionists, scientists, and grandmothers alike. And it is about time that we dispel the myth that eggs are "bad for your cholesterol."

Studies abound showing that the egg is a wholesome and complete protein source, and it is the humble egg that is used for comparison when the quality of other proteins is assessed for their essential amino acid profile. Not only have some studies concluded that eating eggs in the morning is a good way to lose weight, there is also evidence that they can enhance an athlete's game by aiding muscle recovery. Each whole egg contains about six grams of complete protein.

What about high-omega-3 eggs – are they really better? Why can't you just eat the flaxseeds that the chickens are fed, isn't that cheaper? The simplified story is this: humans can eat oils containing EPA (omega-3 from plant sources), which have some protective benefit. But the human body needs to convert the EPA to DHA for use by the brain. Humans are poor converters

of one fat to another; chickens beat us, hands down. So those omega-3 eggs were kindly coddled by chickens who ate the flaxseeds for you and turned their eggs into readily useable DHA.

The yolks of eggs contain cholesterol but they also contain omega-3s to help keep that cholesterol in check. Which means that the yolk of an egg has a neutral effect on your cholesterol level. One of the first steps in controlling cholesterol through diet is to increase omega-3 intake from as many sources as possible, including plant sources like seeds, nuts, and the oils from them, as well as from fish. Given their superior protein and boffo levels of omega-3, you can safely eat one egg three to five times per week.

The best way to cook an egg is to boil or poach it so as not to add any calories or fat. If you are still worried about too much cholesterol, you can get the benefit of eggs by eating egg whites only. Egg whites are a high-quality protein, albeit without the good fat. Packaged egg whites are widely available, and nothing could be easier than opening the carton and pouring them into a hot pan: no waste, low-cal, high-protein.

But perhaps the best thing about eggs is their low cost. A dozen eggs cost about $2 and deliver 72 grams of near-perfect protein along with omega-3 and minerals to spare: 12 grams of protein each for six people. Compare that to one lonely four-ounce pork chop that delivers 22 grams of protein, some minerals but no omega-3s and only the bad saturated fats. The chop costs $2.50 for a portion that feeds only one person. Any way you stir it, eggs win for their affordable, healthy, simple, balanced, and nutritious contribution to your health.

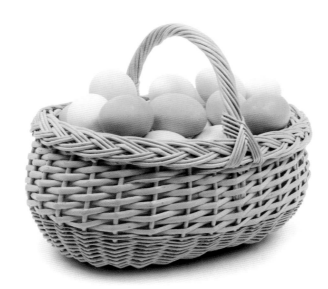

CRAB-STUFFED CREPES

Crepes make excellent use of eggs and are easier to make than pancakes.

	Ingredients	*Benefits*
3	eggs, beaten	leucine for muscle growth and repair
½ cup	whole-wheat flour	mineralized carbohydrate for slow-burning fuel
1 cup	milk	vitamin D-fortified; builds immunity
2 tbsp	butter, melted	butyric acid; balances bowel bacteria
3 x 170-g cans	crabmeat	convenient fish source with high zinc
¾ cup	low-fat plain yogurt	low-fat creaminess
4	green onions, minced	as good as "greens"
2 tbsp	fresh dill, minced	chlorophyll; cleanses liver
½ tsp	white pepper	stimulates saliva; aids digestion
1 clove	garlic, minced	trace minerals
½ cup	low-fat Swiss cheese, grated	concentrated calcium for bones

CREPES: In a large bowl, whisk together eggs, add flour and whisk. Add milk and butter and whisk about 1 minute, until smooth. Refrigerate batter for at least 2 hours and as long as 12 hours before making crepes. To cook crepes, heat cast iron skillet until smoking. Use a paper towel to spread a drop of grapeseed oil just before pouring each crepe. Pour about 3 tbsp of batter into skillet, lightly tip the pan and swirl into a circle; cook until done on one side (it is not necessary to cook crepes on both sides). Wipe pan with paper towel between each crepe. Lay crepes onto clean baking sheet, cooked side down, until ready to fill. (The cooked side has the best presentation and should end up on the outside of the finished product.) Yield: about 12 crepes.

CRAB FILLING: Mix together drained crabmeat, yogurt, green onions, fresh dill, white pepper, and minced garlic. Divide crab mixture among crepes and roll; lay seam side down into a greased lasagna pan. Top with grated cheese. Bake uncovered in preheated 400°F oven 15–20 minutes, until hot. This dish may be refrigerated before baking; remove from refrigerator 30 minutes before baking.

Preparation time: 30–45 minutes Servings: 6

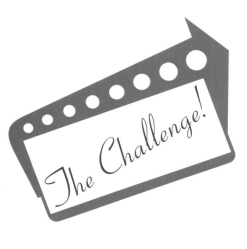

The Challenge!

TAKE A POLL OF 10 friends and ask: "Do eggs affect your cholesterol level?" Record their answers. If you really want to have fun, put some money on it. Share this chapter with a pal and ask him or her to wager a dozen eggs on whether or not people are still operating under outdated information about eggs – kinda like the football pool at the office about which I am ludicrously underinformed.

	YES	NO
1.	☐	☐
2.	☐	☐
3.	☐	☐
4.	☐	☐
5.	☐	☐
6.	☐	☐
7.	☐	☐
8.	☐	☐
9.	☐	☐
10.	☐	☐

FIVE OF CLUBS

CHICKEN: your "go-to" game

Chicken is the most consumed protein in Canada and the United States, and it is growing. There is good reason that we love it so much: chicken carries the flavours of every culture and cuisine beautifully; is a lean, affordable choice; and cooks quickly. Plus, kids like its mild flavour.

From a nutritional perspective, chicken is a powerhouse. Breasts are leaner and a little lower in calories than legs, but legs have more iron and other minerals. Two boneless, skinless thighs or one small chicken breast (either option totals about 100 grams) contain 35 to 50 grams of protein and under 200 calories, providing a good chunk of your protein quota for the day. I prefer thighs because they are more affordable and way juicier; the few extra calories are worth it. However, if you are trying to lose weight, and having chicken two to four times per week, switching to breasts does save a few calories. Either way, whole chicken or pieces can be cooked with the skin on to preserve moisture without adding fat. But don't eat the skin to avoid the majority of the fat.

In a perfect world we would all be able to access affordable, artisan-raised, free range, outdoor grazing chicken but there are downsides to that dream. For instance, we'd be able to get *fresh* chickens only in the summer; they couldn't survive the cold. If I weren't such a city kid I would love to raise them myself (can you sing the *Green Acres* theme song?) but there are laws against raising poultry in most cities and towns, and for good reasons. You could be affecting the health of people and birds nearby. Perhaps the grocery store is a good option, after all?

What are the differences between a conventionally raised and an organic chicken? Certified organic chicken must be fed organic feed. Just as we would choose organic food to fuel our cells and maximize their potential, organic feed produces chicken flesh that tastes superior and is without pesticides. I prefer the deep chickeny flavour, if I have the extra dollars and organic chicken is available to me, I will choose it.

But the biggest myth about conventionally raised chicken in Canada is that it is injected with hormones and steroids. It isn't. Hormones and steroids were banned in Canada back in the 1960s. All commercially raised chickens are free to roam their heated, lighted barns, not caged, and they are safe from airborne disease as well as from predators. *All* Canadian chickens are grain–fed and you can be pretty sure that, no matter where you live, the chicken in your local grocery store is probably a local product.

When I do my final assessment of all the animal proteins available to me at the grocery store, I am perfectly happy with conventionally raised chicken and my conscience is comfortable too.

The best bang for your buck with chicken is to buy it whole:

- When you buy the whole bird, it is one-third the price per pound; when you buy pieces you are paying for the labour that went into cutting it. You can cut the bird into pieces at home in 10 minutes and save 10 bucks! If you eat chicken weekly, that's a lot of cash.
- When you buy pieces, you are throwing out more packaging.
- When you buy a whole bird, you can use the bones for stock and squeeze every ounce of nutrition from one purchase.
- Cutting out the backbone and flattening the bird makes it cook faster, so a whole roaster becomes a weeknight option, with luscious leftovers!

The trouble with barbecuing chicken (beyond the PAHs and HCAs discussed in the Ten of Hearts, but you already know how to fix that!) is that by the time it is cooked through to a safe temperature, the meat is often dry and stringy. The direct and hot external heat just doesn't penetrate the meat evenly. A quick and easy fix is to partially cook it in the microwave and discard any juices. This step will remove some of the bad proteins that create the PAHs and HCAs and cook the chicken halfway while retaining its moisture. A quick drizzle of marinade and an immediate visit to the grill will ensure your healthiest, tastiest helping.

MICROWAVE GRILLED CHICKEN

My favourite smell in the whole world is barbecued chicken. The second I smell it, I am transported back to childhood when summer nights were long and filled with the sounds of kids playing outdoors until the sun set. Nothing but an open flame can create that smell. If you do want to add barbecue sauce, thin your favourite brand with a little water and brush it on just for the last two minutes. This will prevent charring, reduce the salt and sugar you are adding, and yet give you that special smell of summer joy.

	Ingredients	*Benefits*
8	skinless chicken thighs	high-iron, mineral-rich protein
1 tsp	grapeseed oil	heart-protecting fat
4 tbsp	cider vinegar	neutralizes stomach acid
1 tsp	paprika	anticarcinogenic
2 tsp	dried oregano	antibacterial
1 tsp	ground cumin	vitamin E for skin
pinch	cayenne	stimulates metabolism
4 tbsp	bottled barbecue sauce	lycopene; protects prostate
2 tbsp	water	aids fluid balance

Arrange chicken in single layer in a round microwaveable dish or large plate. Microwave chicken on high for 7–10 minutes or until chicken starts to cook. Mix together oil, vinegar, paprika, oregano, cumin, and cayenne in a large bowl. Preheat grill to medium high. Drain juice from chicken and dip each piece into vinegar mixture. (Do not store chicken at this stage; it must be cooked through.) Immediately place chicken on greased grill, close lid, and cook for 10–20 minutes until no longer pink and the internal temperature is 165°F. Turn once or twice

Preparation time: **15 minutes** Servings: **4**

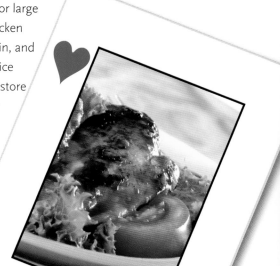

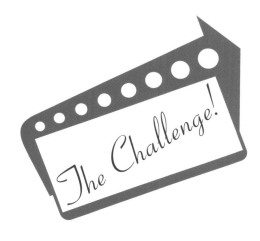

The Challenge!

POLL THE SAME 10 people that you polled about eggs. Ask these 10 people if there are hormones in Canadian chicken. You will be amazed at the misinformation out there.

	YES	NO
1. _____	☐	☐
2. _____	☐	☐
3. _____	☐	☐
4. _____	☐	☐
5. _____	☐	☐
6. _____	☐	☐
7. _____	☐	☐
8. _____	☐	☐
9. _____	☐	☐
10. _____	☐	☐

FOUR OF CLUBS

CHOCOLATE: your best black suit

Finally, some good news: Chocolate is health food! But only dark chocolate (70 percent cocoa), so banish the drugstore chocolate bars and bring on the cocoa powder. Chocolate has about 500 calories per 3.5 ounces (100 grams) so the theme for this food is that a little goes a long way. A one-ounce piece of chocolate is about the size of two fingers. For that amount you get about 166 calories – a small but satisfying snack.

Cocoa powder is the dried solid that is left after most of the cocoa butter is squeezed out of the cacao nut. It is extremely low in calories and extremely high in healthy phytonutrients and flavour. It is what bakers have on hand to make brownies and that you must have on hand to help prevent cancer. The key when choosing a brand is to look for one that does *not* say "Dutch processed"; you want one that says only cocoa powder in its ingredient list. A cocoa powder that is processed using an alkali diminishes the quantity (by half!) of the antioxidants so you can pay less and get more bang for your buck by buying natural cocoa. The initial reason for Dutch processing was to create a smoother flavour with less bitterness (because there are fewer flavonoids), but now that we know that the bitterness is good

for us, bring it on, I say! Often it's the cheaper brands of cocoa that have the single ingredient and that's what you want.

So, how good for you is cocoa anyway?

The antioxidant power of foods is assessed by ORAC value, or Oxygen Radical Absorbance Capacity, which is set by the renowned U.S. National Institute on Aging in the National Institutes of Health (NIH). The website *www. oracvalues.com* lists all the foods that have been tested and their values. The top 10 list consists of spices, some weird stuff – and cocoa powder.

Here is what research has shown so far:

• Free radical damage happens as cells turn over and create waste; it is accelerated when the body is under stress, or in the presence of toxic substances. This simple fact is one of the leading theories on aging and cancer, but we can help the body by providing it with foods high in antioxidants. Think of it as arming every cell with high-quality swords, ammunition, and maps. High-ORAC foods are believed to fight free radical damage. The ORAC value of 100 grams of non–Dutch processed cocoa powder is 80,933; once it is Dutch processed, it drops to 40,200.

- Cocoa powder is a rich source of flavonoids that protect against the clumping together of platelets that can lead to blood clotting.
- Cocoa is high in an amino acid called arginine, which the body requires to make nitric oxide. Nitric oxide causes blood vessels to dilate, resulting in better control over blood flow, inflammation, and blood pressure.
- The cocoa butter in chocolate doesn't appear to adversely affect cholesterol levels.

There are all sorts of new chocolate products that claim to have high ORAC values. My advice is that if you like them and can afford them, by all means, enjoy! If you are disciplined enough to keep your consumption of dark chocolate down to two squares per day, it is a great way to work some healthy treats into your life. A couple of squares of chocolate and three Brazil nuts are ridiculously nutritious and only about 275 calories. You'd be surprised what a filling and satisfying snack these are. My favourite way to include the power of cocoa in the lowest-calorie way is to have a cup of hot cocoa — but not any hot cocoa. I can be found with a cup of ORAC Hot Cocoa in my hand at about 3 p.m. every afternoon from December to March. When I'm staring at sleet and greyness through my window, at least my insides are warm.

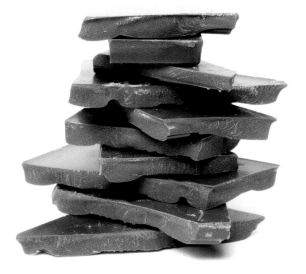

ORAC HOT COCOA

This beverage is so rich you feel as if you are having a decadent treat, yet it is the most nutrient-packed 60 calories per mug that you will find. It is important not to skip the maple syrup, which keeps the cocoa (and therefore the antioxidants) in solution rather than sinking to the bottom. Mixing the maple syrup in with the cocoa also creates a foamy top, a flourish that you would pay a barista way too much for.

Ingredients — *Benefits*

	Ingredients	Benefits
1 tbsp	pure maple syrup	nutrient-dense sweetener
1 tbsp	cocoa powder (not Dutch processed)	high-ORAC food
pinch	cinnamon	high-ORAC spice
¾–1½ cup	boiling water	pure hydration
¼ cup	low-fat milk	calcium; protects tooth enamel

Use a fork to blend together maple syrup and cocoa powder; stir vigorously until completely blended. Add boiling water to fill your cup two-thirds full, stir thoroughly with fork. Top with milk.

Preparation time: **2 minutes** Servings:1

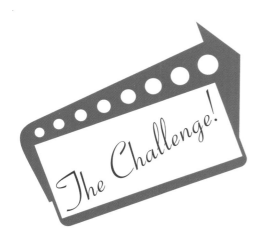

TASTE-TEST MULTIPLE BRANDS OF chocolate to find one that you like. Each brand has its own blend using varying amounts of cocoa butter and added ingredients, so you may have to go through a few to hit the sweet spot. Some brands have added fruits and/or nuts; just go by your personal preference.

Doing this challenge with a friend is more fun, because you can test each other. Don't be influenced by packaging or preconceived notions about the product. Look for a chocolate that has at least 70 percent cocoa to obtain the health benefits. Go for the highest percentage that you can before the bitterness (of the chocolate not the fact that you can't have drugstore candy bars any more!) stops you from enjoying it. Try at least three different brands.

Taste-testing steps:

- Set one square of each chocolate on a plate.
- Assess with your eyes first. The samples should be slightly shiny, and dark and deep in colour.
- Assess with your nose. The smell should appeal to you and be more chocolatey and less cocoa buttery.
- Taste with your entire tongue, spreading the chocolate around as it melts, breathing through your nose to mix in air, the way a wine taster would. Is the taste too sweet or too bitter?
- Feel whether the texture appeals to you. Does it feel waxy or slippery? The chocolate should melt and spread without squeaking on your teeth.
- Score each sample on a scale of 1 to 10.

Now, find a way to work chocolate into your life, each and every day. You are welcome!

THREE OF CLUBS

SPICES AND HERBS: Ancient wisdom meets New Age science

My mother treated our ear infections with garlic juice and her grandmother may have used willow bark tea for pain and honey for skin infections. Neither knew that the future would prove their techniques bang on. We now know that garlic is antibacterial and antimicrobial, thus its effectiveness in our ears. We also know that the formula for aspirin, the single most used blood thinner in North America, was invented using that very same willow bark.

Honey now has science behind it as a more potent antibiotic than penicillin. We are just beginning to understand *why* these traditional remedies work but there is no doubt that they *do* work!

The goal of pharmacological research is to isolate useful chemicals so that they can be recreated and sythesized in the lab. But it just may be that when you isolate you also remove something that is fundamental to effectiveness. For instance, does your body use vitamin C supplements as effectively as when you eat an entire orange? Or is there something in the orange that makes the vitamin C more potent, more effective, or more usable by your body? Visual, taste, and smell sensors are our way of discerning what is consumable. We are designed to understand our surroundings. A red berry is easily spotted in a green forest, its smell draws us in and its taste is sweet and pleasant, which sends the same signal to human and animal alike: *Eat me.*

Traditional Indian Ayurvedic medicine used a treasure trove of spices before scientists even considered testing them for efficacy. Cinnamon is an easy spice to eat daily and it has been a proven tool in the fight against diabetes and high blood pressure. A half-teaspoon per day was all it took in one study to improve glucose tolerance and protect blood vessels. Cinnamon is showing promise in some studies for controlling cholesterol as well. There is only one simple, tasty way to find out. Sprinkle it on everything from peanut butter to hot cocoa to oatmeal.

Eugenol, which is a volatile oil found in clove

oil, is used in dentistry for its anti-inflammatory, analgesic effect. A drop of clove oil rubbed on a sore spot in the mouth soothes the pain. Herbs and spices are ridiculously high in antioxidant activity, as you have seen on the ORAC website. It is truly a shame that the average North American palate is so bland, because the most intensely flavoured herbs and spices are the ones that fight hardest for us. Our tongues have adapted to over-saltiness but cringe at many spice flavours.

Curcumin is the principal compound in turmeric, which is the spice that lends a yellow colour to curry powder. Turmeric is under serious investigation as a cancer treatment. It appears to be curcumin's ability to encourage apoptosis in cells that is so beneficial. Apoptosis is the message within each and every cell that tells it when it's time to call it quits. Cancer cells are often missing this message or are able to ignore it, which is thought to be the reason they proliferate so vigorously. They are like the loud obnoxious drunks at a party who refuse to take the hint. Curcumin is the bouncer with the muscle to toss out cancer cells.

Cancer is much easier to prevent than to treat. If something as delicious as curry can help me stay cancer-free, it seems like a good thing to include in my roster. Some evidence points to turmeric's enhanced potency when cooked or consumed with oils, which is what traditional curry cooks do. (I love it when wonderful things happen seemingly by accident!) The proper Indian technique is to heat the oil, and then stir in the spices to open up their flavours before adding other ingredients to the pot. As a shortcut you can use one of the better bottled curry sauces that are prepared in this traditional fashion, but check the labels for sodium content and that they contain real butter rather than vegetable ghee or margarine.

Here are some tips for working curry spices in to your life:

- Turmeric won't be noticed in a spaghetti sauce and adds a certain *je ne sais quoi* to chili.
- Turmeric is tasty in egg salad, made with yogurt instead of mayo.
- Steam cauliflower, broccoli, and/or carrots or boil potatoes or sweet potatoes, then stir fry with a tablespoon of butter and a tablespoon of curry powder or turmeric.
- Bake whole sweet potatoes in the oven until soft, then peel off the skins and mash with turmeric and olive oil.
- Spice cake is enhanced with a pinch of turmeric and a pinch of cayenne pepper, on top of the sweet spices that are already there.

DOROWAT

(ETHIOPIAN CHICKEN AND CHICKPEAS)

Made with a number of the spices on the Top 10 ORAC list, this version of the sweet
stew that can be found in Ethiopia is a powerhouse of antioxidants.

Ingredients		*Benefits*
28-oz can	crushed tomatoes	lycopene; anticarcinogenic
¾ cup	dry red wine	heart-healthy polyphenols
¼ cup	paprika	capsaicin; anti-inflammatory
1 tbsp	red chili pepper flakes	capsaicin; anti-inflammatory
1 tbsp	ground turmeric	curcumin; boosts immunity
1 tbsp	grapeseed oil	heart-healthy fat
	medium onion, minced	flavour-rich fibre
2	garlic cloves, minced	allicin; fights cold virus
2 tbsp	ginger root, grated	aids digestion
1 tsp	ground nutmeg	high ORAC value
1 tsp	ground cloves	analgesic; digestive aid
1 tsp	ground allspice	high ORAC value
1 tsp	cinnamon	regulates blood pressure
1 lb	skinless chicken thighs	lean protein
28-oz can	chickpeas, drained	high-protein, high-fibre legume

In a large bowl, combine tomatoes, ½ cup of the red wine, paprika, chili pepper flakes, and
turmeric, and set aside. Warm a large deep pot over medium-high heat. Add oil, and cook onion
for about 5 minutes. Add garlic and grated ginger, cook for 1 more minute. Stir in the spices then
add chicken pieces and brown for 2–4 minutes per side. Pour tomato mixture over chicken and
bring to boiling; reduce heat. Cover and simmer about 30 minutes. Stir in remaining ¼ cup dry
red wine and drained chickpeas. Simmer uncovered for about 15 minutes.

Preparation time: 25 minutes Servings: 12

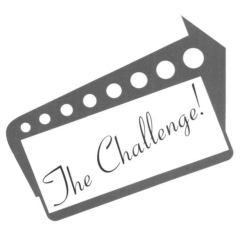

The Challenge!

FIND SOMEONE OVER 80 years old and have a conversation about traditional remedies. It will be a fascinating topic for you but perhaps even more rewarding for them to be able to share their knowledge. Find out what they used to do when their kids had colic or how they treated scuffed knees. Ask what they did/do to fight colds or find out if they have secret poultices for fever. Document their answers and give them a framed copy as a gift – a warm way to contribute to the preservation of ancient knowledge for future generations.

TWO OF CLUBS

Breathing is the most basic thing that we do to keep us alive. The perils of drawing in smoggy breath are well documented, as are those of smoking, but the airborne dangers in our impeccably clean houses can often be overlooked. It may be too big a step for you to get rid of your regular cleaning products (which are toxic, which you do inhale, and which do have a negative impact on your health, particularly on your liver), so let's start small. (But if you can throw out your cleaning products, go ahead!)

There are two things you need to remove from your home that will improve your air quality immeasurably: non-stick skillets and, ironically, air fresheners. Non-stick coatings contain a chemical called PTFE (polytetrafluoroethylene), which has been found in human blood from one coast to the other, in rich and poor alike. Long-term exposure to PTFE has been identified as carcinogenic, and it never breaks down in the body or the environment. Some defenders say that this coating is safe as long as it is not overheated. And by overheated they mean nothing above medium. These skillets can get to 500 degrees Fahrenheit on medium-high heat in less than two minutes when empty. At that temperature, everyone agrees that they emit a gas that is dangerous when inhaled. (The flakes themselves may pass right through the human system, but it is suspected that the scratches in the pan actually allow more gas to escape!)

Committing to using only medium heat won't work for most of us hurried chefs, and inevitably the pan will get scratched, which only increases the risk over time. There are two easy solutions. The first is to replace your non-stick pan with any one of a line of skillets made with ceramic coatings, often sold with such descriptors as "healthy chef" and "green cookware" (these are in the $60 to $120 range). These coatings are safe to over 500 degrees and one good skillet will last for a decade or two.

The cheaper alternative is a cast iron skillet. A good cast iron skillet costs under $20 ($4 if you pick one up at a yard sale or thrift shop) and will last generations. Even a rusty one can be brought back to life. The best thing about a cast iron skillet from a chef's perspective is that it can get to a really high temperature quickly and hold that temperature, which allows for a terrific sear and creates a wonderful colour on everything from meat to mushrooms. The best thing about a cast iron skillet from a nutritionist's perspective is that it enhances the iron uptake in foods, which can be crucial for a vegetarian or any woman of child-bearing age. You get more or less iron depending upon what goes in the pan and how it is cared for: acidic foods, more iron; well-seasoned pan, less iron.

The trick to making your cast iron pan a lifelong friend is a simple preparatory step called "seasoning." Give it a good rinse and scrape under hot running water and a good rub with a steel wool cleaning pad (do not use soap) to remove as much rust as you can (or the top layer of a new pan). Place the clean pan on a burner over high heat to dry. This is how you will dry the pan every time you use it. Now turn off the heat and pour a teaspoon of cooking oil into the pan, swirl or rub with paper towel. Pour off any remaining oil. Sprinkle with a tablespoon of salt, which will act as a grit to remove any old skuzz

or rust. Dump residue and run the pan under the tap. Place back on the burner over high heat and allow to dry. The skillet is now seasoned and will be just as non-stick as your old PFTE-emitting pan.

Clearing the air of air fresheners is even easier. The phthalates in the perfumes in these and other cleaning, hair, and skin products are suspected of damaging the liver, kidneys, and lungs. Phthalates are hormone disrupters that mimic sex hormones and are thought to increase cancer risk. Europe has already banned them. The best way to clear the air is to open a window as often as possible, and it doesn't cost you a penny. Or you could make your own air freshener. Pour a quarter cup or so of vinegar mixed with the same amount of water into a small ceramic bowl and add a tablespoon or so of spices such as cinnamon sticks, cardamom pods, or whole cloves. Place this bowl in front of, on top of, or near a heat source or sunny window on each level of your house. As the vinegar evaporates, it will acidify the air and kill airborne mould, and as the water evaporates it will carry the scent of the spices with it. For strong cooking smells, simmer an open pot of water containing the mixture on the stove and turn on a fan. Cheap, easy, fresh, and carcinogen-free.

CAST IRON CORN BREAD

This bread is nothing like the dry salty stuff that comes in a package. It's great as a starch side dish or served for a snack with cheese and pure maple syrup.

Ingredients

		Benefits
1½ cups	yellow cornmeal	lutein for eyes
1½ cups	whole-wheat flour	fibre; combats metabolic syndrome
1 tbsp	baking powder	avoids baker's yeast, a common allergen
1 tsp	baking soda	alkali; aids digestion
¾ tsp	sea salt	trace minerals
3 tbsp	butter	more digestible than margarine
1 cup	frozen corn	thiamin; for brain function
2½ cups	buttermilk	lower-fat dairy
¼ cup	honey	antibacterial sweetener
3	eggs	vitamin E for glowing skin
3	egg whites	lean protein for muscle maintenance
1 tbsp	grapeseed oil	best fat for high heat

In a very large bowl, mix together cornmeal and whole-wheat flour. Stir in baking powder, baking soda, and salt. Combine butter and corn in a separate bowl, and heat in microwave until butter is melted. Whisk in buttermilk, honey, eggs, and egg whites. Pour buttermilk mixture into cornmeal mixture and stir to mix.

Preheat a large cast iron skillet over high heat for 2–3 minutes. When skillet is steaming, pour in grapeseed oil and wipe it up the sides of the pan with paper towel (be careful, the pan is hot!). Quickly pour cornmeal mixture into the pan and let it bake on the bottom over medium heat for 2–3 minutes while oven preheats. Bake at 400°F on the top shelf of the oven until firm, approximately 20–30 minutes.

Preparation time: **20 minutes** Servings: **24**

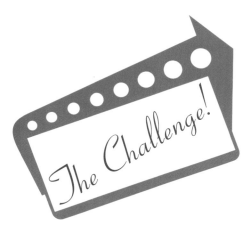
The Challenge!

NOW THAT YOU KNOW what the health costs are for air fresheners, let's do the math on how much your air fresheners are costing you in real dollars each year.

Plug-in holder	$_____
x ___ number of holders	$_____
Total A:	**$_____**
Cost of refills	$_____
x ___ number of refills/year	$_____
Total B:	**$_____**
Cost of other room/carpet/furniture sprays for one month	$_____
x 12 months (**Total C**):	$_____
Grand total, A + B + C:	**$_____**

Take this money and treat yourself to something nice with it or donate it to an environmental organization.

PART 4

The Diamonds are the gems in life, the highest, brightest peak in our hierarchy of needs. This is where we maximize the skills that can make our lives better. Some of these are the tricks that your infant and your dog employ daily. But don't discount them as lightweight. There is evidence that busting stress through listening, laughter, and stretching can save your heart just as much as eating fish and running a marathon. Some of us (me!) need to work a little smarter at this end to pull it all together without burning out.

It is easy – once you learn that eating dessert, managing holidays, and stopping to hear the birds is as crucial to your overall health as remembering to eat a high-quality breakfast. However, participating in life's daily adventures without being overwhelmed, overworked, and outplayed is a balancing act that can be difficult to manage. And it's not just your body that needs to be maintained and well fed. You won't make much progress if you don't have good mental health, and that includes everything from stress management to the benefits of helping others. The game, you see, has always been played in your own head.

ACE OF DIAMONDS

VITAMINS AND SUPPLEMENTS: Pill power or expensive pee?

There are experts who swear by megadoses of vitamins and experts who believe we should be able to get all we need from food. I'm somewhere in between.

If all of our food were locally and organically grown *and* we ate two or three times the average amount of vegetables North Americans currently consume, then maybe our diets would serve us sufficiently. If we had less stress to contend with and no smog or toxic cleansers to inhale, we could get by on just the food we ate. If we expected to live only to 45 years of age, we could continue to happily count only on food to preserve our health.

But the truth is that we eat sub-par foods and not enough of the good stuff; we are chronic stress bunnies living in smoggy cities or pesticide-sprayed countryside; and we want every healthy year that we can get out of this life. If a multi-vitamin can counteract these shortcomings, why wouldn't I give myself a fighting chance? And Statistics Canada tells us that 70 percent of our kids do not consume even the minimum of five servings of fruits and vegetables each day. We all

need to "fill in the blanks" with a reliable multi-vitamin to be sure that we are getting the small but crucial micronutrients and co-factors that may be missing from our busy lives.

However, the vitamin naysayers have a point, too. They counter that the average consumer has no way of knowing whether labels are accurate or reliable. And there have been cases where mega-doses of nutrients have been later found to be dangerous. Vitamin E, for instance, was the wunderkind of the 1990s, and later studies showed it to be a factor in over-thinning the blood or interacting with medications when the synthetic form was taken at doses above 400 IU per day. Folic acid, still believed to be the best way to prevent neural tube defects in fetuses, may stimulate the growth of existing cancerous or precancerous cells that would otherwise remain stable. For that reason, it is recommended that no one should be taking more than 400 micrograms (mcg) of folic acid as a supplement for an extended period of time. You see how complex this can get? That's because food is meant to be complex and any time you isolate one nutrient, you affect the actions that it can take, so getting as much nutrition as possible from food is advisable.

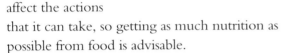

The simple fact is that food delivers a well-designed package of both macro- and micronutrients, fibre, and water – all the elements needed to sustain and enhance life. That said, there are exceptions to every rule. Some people's bodies require more of a specific nutrient. For instance, a few years ago, I experienced an unusual symptom: a burning sensation on my tongue. No doctor or dentist could explain it. Even more baffling, it wasn't constant but, for no apparent reason whatsoever, it would sneak up on me throughout the day. I would wake up feeling fine and go to bed wishing I could rip out my tongue. The diagnosis was "burning mouth syndrome" and the Internet was rife with completely unhelpful, useless "information" and "tips." I was almost resigned to living with it (and paying a shrink to help me deal with the depression) when I asked a colleague for her opinion.

Aileen has her PhD in immunology, is crazy-smart, and works in the biochemical nutrition field (also known as ortho-molecular medicine). "Oh, that," she said. "Try B_1."

She was right: I was B_1 deficient! (Each of the B vitamins has its own job to do but most factor into the metabolization of carbohydrates and the ability to manage stress. So, as the Type A child of a long line of diabetics having a B_1 deficiency made sense.) Problem solved and a convert created! There is no way of knowing why this happened to me. But, for a chef, this affliction is about the worst thing that *could* happen. I rarely have flare-ups now but I do notice that they occur during times of higher stress. As long as I have a few B_1 pills daily I am right as rain. I would urge anyone with mysterious health problems to contact a naturopath or nutritionist who specializes in orthomolecular health. They may be able to safely treat weird conditions that confound your doctor.

So, if you are convinced that supplements do have a role to play, the next question is what is safe and what is necessary? Let's start with the basics that you've already read about here:

OMEGA-3 FROM FISH OIL	1,000–2,000 MILLIGRAMS PER DAY
MAGNESIUM	100–400 MILLIGRAMS PER DAY
VITAMIN D	1,000 IU MILLIGRAMS PER DAY

Add to this a multivitamin that should have no more than:

VITAMIN A	4,000 IU
BETA CAROTENE	6,000 IU
FOLIC ACID	400 mcg

Your doctor or naturopath may recommend other supplements to help with specific issues (for instance, calcium to strengthen bones).

Choose your multivitamin based on what you can afford. Most of the major brands and the generic brands in Canada have good formulations. If there are additional marketing banners touting added extracts, be sure that the claims are based on solid, third-party evidence. Much of the research I have seen so far in this burgeoning industry is pointing toward the fact that you may be better off eating foods like cranberries and drinking green tea than taking their extracts in pill form! With the possible exception of probiotics added to your multivitamin. Since these are coated to make them stable through the stomach, they remain viable until they reach the bowel where they are most useful. Take your multivitamin with food in the morning or at lunch so you can make the best use of the fuel. If you have tummy trouble, look for a liquid and take smaller amounts more frequently.

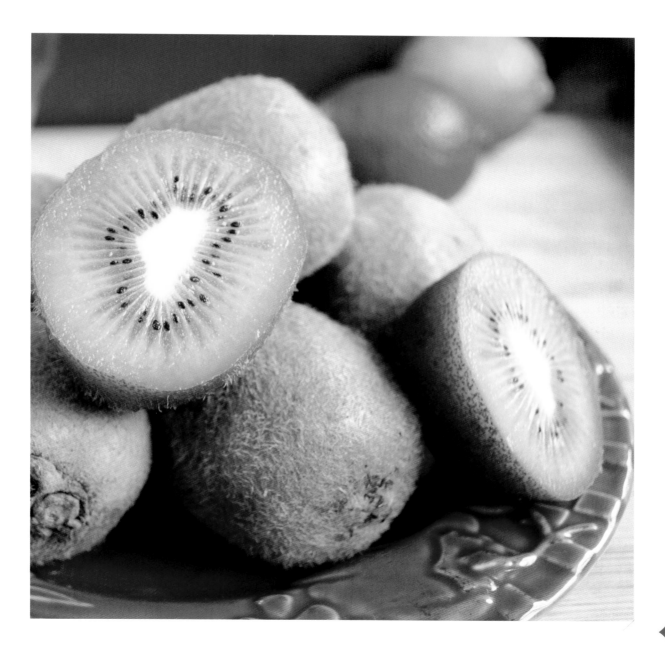

KIWI SALSA

Vitamin C is one of the nutrients best obtained from food to the extent possible, because supplements may not be as beneficial. Kiwi fruit is one of the highest sources of vitamin C available. (The skins, if you can stand the furry texture, are edible and contain excellent fibre.) This salsa is a treat as a dip for corn chips, but is also delicious to dress up any fish or chicken dish. Simply spread it on after baking or grilling.

Ingredients		*Benefits*
6	kiwi fruit, peeled and chopped	vitamin C
2 tsp	mint, chopped	vitamins C and A
1 4–5 oz can	jalapenos, chopped, drained	capsaicin; stimulates circulation
1	lime, juiced (or 2 tbsp bottled juice)	vitamin C
2 tbsp	extra virgin olive oil	assists uptake of fat-soluble vitamins
1 tbsp	honey	trace minerals
1 tbsp	balsamic vinegar	alkalizing; aids digestion
	salt and pepper, to taste	

Toss together all ingredients and allow to sit at room temperature for about 1 hour before serving. Salsa keeps well in fridge for up to 3 days.

Preparation time: 15 minute Servings: 16

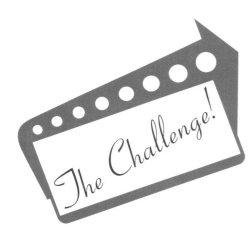

The Challenge!

CHOOSE YOUR MULTIVITAMIN WISELY by holding it up against this list, which outlines the minimums and maximums according to the latest and safest research. Keep in mind that no one pill can cover off all that you may need without becoming too large to swallow, and an extra separate supplement for some nutrients may be needed.

No more than: *My multivitamin has:*

4,000 IU vitamin A

6,000 IU beta carotene

100 IU natural-source vitamin E

400 mcg (0.4 mg) folic acid

Most other nutrients are in small amounts and/or are water soluble (so you'll pee them out) and have no toxicity effects.

Also look for these nutrients if you aren't getting enough of them from food:

Omega-3 from fish oil (see Jack of Hearts)

1,000-2,000 milligrams per day

Vitamin D (see King of Clubs)

1000 IU per day

Magnesium (see Queen of Hearts)

100-400 milligrams per day

Probiotics such as acidophilus and bifidus and prebiotics such as FOS (fructooligosaccharides)

KING OF DIAMONDS

DOLLARS AND SENSE: What's the cost of all this health?

———————

I don't deny that it can cost money to join a gym, buy vitamins, and eat fresh, organic food. But there are a few arguments that bring these decisions into better focus.

What is the hard cost to your health if you don't protect it now? Preventable illness is extremely costly even with universal health care. Over-the-counter remedies for cold and flu and pain do add up. The loss of a job due to health problems can set you back years in savings. Medications are not covered by most provincial healthcare plans unless you are a senior. Many cancer treatment drugs become out-of-pocket expenses if you don't have a private plan and even then . . . need I go on?

What is the cost to our healthcare system as a result of people not making better choices? We live in a country that takes care of everyone, which means that we have help when we need it, but wouldn't it be better if we didn't partake unnecessarily? Doesn't it save us all in taxes if a little education keeps more of us out of the hospital?

Haven't we got the equation wrong when choosing good food? It would help to see the equation as cents per nutrient, and what these nutrients can do for you, rather than as cents per (often empty) calorie. Buying (cheap) bad food just because it fills you up may have been a useful strategy when food was scarce but it simply isn't valid anymore.

Where else are we spending our money? Our priorities seem to be the next gaming system or mobile phone. These toys and trinkets are wonderful and I am an avid user of them but not at the cost of what goes into my body. For $1,000 I can choose between a new laptop and the finest fish and chicken three times per week for my whole family for a year. My clunky old laptop is working just fine. Thanks anyway. And there are ways to stretch that $1,000 even further. Beans and tofu are less expensive than even the cheapest cut of meat. Taking the $3 or $4 per day that many of us spend on store-bought coffee could cover the cost of supplements for the whole family.

I was in a grocery store recently and watched a young mother shopping for herself and her toddler. She carefully scanned for sales on each shelf and read labels dutifully. She went to the reduced bin and scooped up asparagus, a mango, and red peppers that had been on the regular shelves only seconds before. Then she went to the fish counter and asked for fish heads (presumably to make soup). Her choice of the largest bag of brown rice probably cut into her weekly budget but it will last her a year. The dried beans that she chose cost less than $1.50

and were enough for at least 10 meals for her and her daughter.

What she did not do was agonize over the 10 extra cents that it cost to buy whole-grain bread over the white. She also did not buy any packaged sweets or snacks. At the risk of appearing to be a stalker, I followed her to the checkout counter. I wanted to know what her purchases cost. No kidding, the fruits and veggies were less than a dollar, as was the fish. I wanted to hug her, but that might have gotten me arrested so I didn't push it. But I saved her story to prove that healthy eating can be inexpensive.

As often as possible in *Ace Your Health* I have given high-end and low-end options. The rest is up to you.

RED LENTIL AND SWEET POTATO SOUP

You can feed a family of eight on $3.76 with a soup of high-protein lentils, nutrition-packed sweet potatoes, and onions. Cheese is optional and will cost a bit extra.

	Ingredients	*Benefits*
1 tsp	butter	healthy saturated fats
1	onion, chopped	sulphur; combats heart disease
2	small sweet potatoes, cubed	vitamin A for eyes
4 cups	chicken or vegetable broth	high-nutrient, low-calorie
4 cups	water	supports kidney function
2 cups	red lentils	plant-based protein
1 tbsp	dried basil	phytonutrients; protect eyes
2 tsp	dried red chili peppers	enhances metabolism
½ tsp	black pepper	stimulates digestion
2 tbsp	molasses	high in minerals
8 tbsp	grated cheddar cheese (optional)	calcium for bones

Warm a large pot over medium-high heat and melt butter. Add onions and sweet potatoes; stir. Add broth and water; add lentils. Bring to a boil, turn down to simmer and cover. Let simmer for 20 minutes. Stir in basil, chili peppers, pepper and molasses. Grate cheese if using and serve at the table.

Preparation time: 25 minutes Servings: 8 to 10

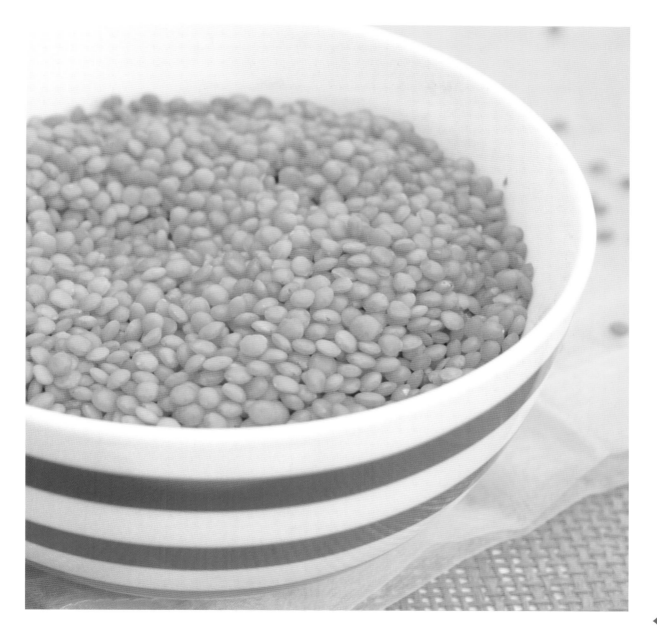

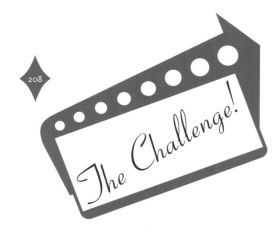

The Challenge!

FIND FREE MONEY. HERE is a list of things that you could do to find an estimated $2 per day that you could reinvest in your health. Many of these tips help save the planet too!

- Avoid coffee shops; bring a Thermos.
- Reduce unnecessary restaurant meals.
- Forgo store-bought treats and bake at home.
- Buy one less or one cheaper bottle of wine or make your own.
- Car pool or take public transit.
- Use coupons.
- Read the newspaper online.
- Turn your thermostat down a couple of degrees and/or turn it down overnight.
- Share books or use the local library.
- Use reusable cups and containers instead of plastic sandwich bags.
- Keep tea in your desk. Boil water in the microwave or the lunchroom kettle at work.
- Grow your own flowers.
- Press or dry flowers, so you can enjoy them through the winter.
- Shovel your own driveway.
- Can your own veggies and fruit.
- Make your own jams.
- Have cocktails at home rather than at a bar.
- Use only your bank's ATMs.
- Buy spices, teas, and candies in bulk.
- Say no to impulse buys.
- Order tap water in restaurants and don't buy bottled water.
- Do your own nails.
- Buy clothes, dishes, and furniture at thrift stores.

- Cut out useless features on your cell phone or cable TV.
- Pay bills on time to avoid late fees or interest penalties.
- Do only full loads of laundry.
- Hang clothes outside to dry in summer or in the basement in winter.
- Run the dishwasher only when full.
- Fix leaky faucets.
- Turn off lights.
- Hem your own pants and skirts.

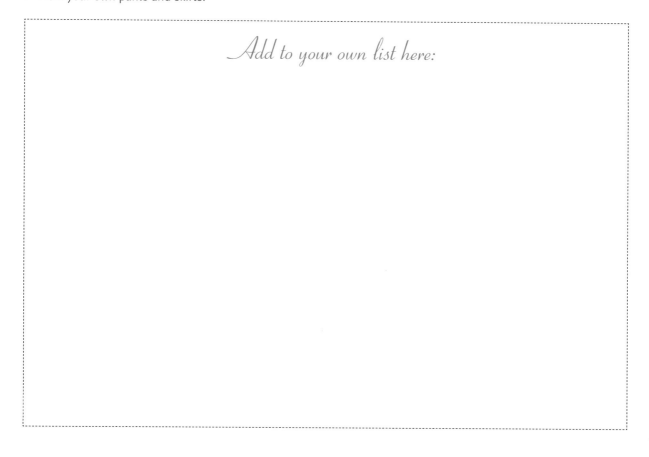

Add to your own list here:

QUEEN OF DIAMONDS

STRETCHING: Never stretch the truth

There are two ways to stretch: the micro way that you do to uncramp your muscles when you are forced into awkward positions for long periods of time (like writing a book, say) and the macro way, which is an activity done to strengthen muscles and increase flexibility. There are darned good reasons to do both, but the main one is that it feels good. Watch your dog or cat any day of the week and you will see the joy on their faces as they stretch. Stretching can be beneficial even when it is as simple as a cat arching her back. Or that bum up, front paws on the ground, long, slow lunge a lazy dog does when you say it is time to go for a walk on a rainy day.

If you did nothing other than this each and every day, you would notice increased flexibility, and when muscles are more flexible everyday tasks become easier and there is less chance of injury. I have seen people whose bodies are so tight that they have pulled muscles just reaching up to close the car trunk!

Regular stretching provides the following benefits:

- **Increased range of motion**. When the muscles supporting your joints are flexible, the body can move with ease in different directions with greater stability. With a healthy range of motion and stability, you're less likely to fall or lose your balance. Slipping on the ice or down the stairs may seem like a mundane mishap but such accidents can wreck lives.

- **Improved circulation.** Circulation factors into every process that the body does, from keeping you warm at rest to recovering from a workout. Who doesn't want their heart to work more efficiently?

- **Increased body awareness.** If we take time to focus on our muscles while we stretch, we become in tune with what's going on in our bodies. With conscious body awareness, we're less likely to overeat, to strain muscles, or to push our body beyond its limits.

- **Relieved stress.** Perhaps the most important argument for stretching is that it relieves stress simply by reducing muscle tension. The biofeedback to the brain helps calm the stress hormones. The Jack of Diamonds has more information on this subject.

We humans tend to carry most of our tension in the large muscle groups like thighs, hips, and lower back, as well as our calves, shoulders, and neck. The Internet is rife with videos and photos on how to stretch. Start small and implement these few tips:

- Warm up before you stretch to get your blood flowing. A quick three-minute walk on the spot, dance, or sprint up a couple of flights of stairs is all it takes. Rather than stretching *before* you exercise, do it after; it's a great way to cool down, speed recovery, and help release the stress hormones of a heart-pounding run.
- Hold each stretch for at least 30 seconds; it takes that long to let the muscle fibre relax.
- Do not bounce or force yourself into a stretch. This can tear your muscle tissue and cause it to scar, which will only tighten you further.
- You want to feel a nice tension, not pain. Over time, you will be able to stretch further.
- Breathing is vital. Take a deep breath and exhale while trying to stretch a little further.

By far, the most interesting and popular type of stretching is yoga. Accessing this life-altering activity couldn't be easier. There are videos, webinars, and classes available everywhere and it isn't all crunchy granola woo-woo. There are several types of yoga. My favourite is slow and restful Hatha yoga, but there's also the more active Ashtanga yoga and Bikram (hot) yoga. Any form of yoga practice is beneficial: from lowering blood pressure to reducing the symptoms of asthma and osteoarthritis, depression, and lower-back pain. Studies have found a positive impact on the inflammatory markers of heart disease and up to a 20 percent regression in the hardening of the arteries. Prison inmates who do yoga have shown a lower occurrence of psychiatric episodes.

It is hard to say whether it is the stress relief of deep breathing and taking a moment to slow down or the actual stretching that makes such a huge difference. Who cares? If all it takes is an hour or two per week to reap such huge benefits in such a pleasant way, I am in!

EASY FOCACCIA

While you are stretching the dough in this recipe, watch how it relaxes under your fingers. You will notice that it is easier when the dough is at room temperature and not just out of the fridge. A small square of this bread makes a great accompaniment to a soup or salad lunch. Leftovers are terrific cut into cubes, rebaked at 300°F and left to dry. Store these in an airtight container for up to three weeks and use a few as croutons in soup or salad.

Ingredients

		Benefits
1	standard premade whole-wheat pizza dough	whole grains; stabilize insulin
1–3 tsp	extra virgin olive oil	moisturizes skin
¼ cup	grated Parmesan cheese	reduces need for salt
1 tbsp	dried rosemary	traditional remedy for nasal congestion
1	garlic clove, minced	sulphur for strong heart
pinch	sea salt, to taste	trace minerals
1 tbsp	white chia seeds	highest-quality fibre

If dough is frozen thaw on counter. Leave at room temperature in an oiled bowl in the oven away from drafts to rise for 1–6 hours. The process is extremely forgiving so take as little or as long as you need. Lay dough on a cookie sheet and lightly oil your hands. Gently stretch dough from the centre outward, using the flat palm of your hands. Hold for a few seconds and don't bounce! Move the dough as close to the edges of the pan as you can. Have patience, stretching the dough out takes time.

Heat oven to 400°F. Sprinkle dough with cheese, rosemary, garlic, sea salt, and chia. Bake for 15–18 minutes until brown. Let cool slightly and cut into 24 squares. Feel free to spice it up with crushed red pepper flakes.

Preparation time: 10 minutes Servings: 24

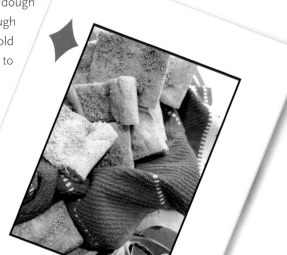

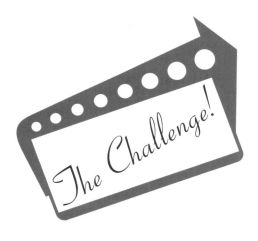
The Challenge!

FIND A WAY TO fit some kind of stretching into your day this week. It could be as simple as a five-minute arched-back cat stretch or as committed as a new yoga class. You can purchase a yoga DVD, or go on *www.clearspaceonline.com* or on YouTube and imitate a simple yoga posture like the warrior pose. I admit to using my daughter's Wii Fit to walk me through a few poses if I am really pressed for time. Feedback from the animated trainer gives me an extra nudge of motivation.

Keep a daily tally of every five-minute bout of stretching you do this week and write the total here:

	DAILY STRETCHING TIME	IF YOUR WEEKLY TOTAL IS . . .	YOUR GRADE IS . . .
MONDAY		LESS THAN 35 MINUTES	F
TUESDAY		35–60 MINUTES	C
WEDNESDAY		60–120 MINUTES	C+
THURSDAY		120–180 MINUTES	B
FRIDAY		180–240 MINUTES	B+
SATURDAY		240–300 MINUTES	A
SUNDAY		OVER 300 MINUTES	A+

JACK OF DIAMONDS

STRESS: Breathing down the neck of this killer

———

We all experience stress. It is neither good nor bad, it simply exists and is necessary. It is life's inbox that makes us get out of bed in the morning, knowing that there is something that *must be done*. Oddly enough, without that sense of purpose, life would be more stressful.

The *most* stressed-out people are those who have the *least* control over their lives. Those at the bottom of the corporate structure are most susceptible. They perform never-ending tasks: another stack of letters is always coming to the letter carrier, the phone will continue to ring for the receptionist, and the people will continue to wait, often grumpily in the cold, for the bus driver to open the doors. If you do this kind of job you probably suffer more from stress than your CEO.

According to the American Institute of Stress, 75 to 90 percent of all visits to primary care physicians are for stress-related complaints or conditions. Health Canada says that employees who are under sustained stress have three times more heart and back problems; five times more cancers; two to three times more mental health issues; and are two times more likely to have substance abuse issues.

Clearly we need to do something about our stress. To get a handle on stress, it is helpful to divide it into two piles – neither one smells pretty but at least you know where to start. The first pile consists of all the things that you can do nothing about like death, taxes, and in-laws. The second pile contains the things that you have a hope of changing, like health, homework, and job status. It soon becomes clear that most of what causes stress is in the pile that is changeable. This is great news because you have the power to lower your stress levels directly by altering any and everything that causes stress. Once you know this is so, you just have to gather your support network and act! If taking action is not possible in the short run, your next best bet is to alter how you perceive the situations that cause you stress.

The best way to handle stress is to change the things that you can and learn to accept the things that you can't. But acceptance doesn't mean throwing in the towel; it means developing coping strategies.

- Take a meditation class or course. Meditation can lower blood pressure and stress hormone levels. There are many methods and approaches; just do a little research to find the right fit.
- Learn how to breathe properly (see this week's challenge).
- Sing out loud. Big (proper) breath in and hold it, then let it out slowly while you hold a note. The sound doesn't have to be beautiful. Anyone can do this.

(The exception is my husband: we let him sing only when he is alone or it causes the rest of us undue stress!) Singing also causes a soothing, rhythmic vibration in your chest, a lot like the purring of a cat.
- Since you're already singing, why not listen to some upbeat tunes? I love all sorts of music but for me, in times of stress, it's Miley Cyrus's song "The Climb" that puts a smile on my face and opens my heart to the possibilities of life.
- There are many herbal remedies for stress. Passion-flower drops found at health food stores can be very powerful. Just make sure that your doctor and pharmacist know that you are taking them: they may interact with any drugs that you are on.

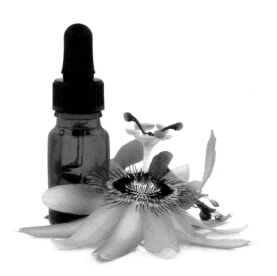

WEEKNIGHT TURKEY DINNER

Tryptophan is an amino acid that is the precursor to serotonin, which is the "feel good" neurotransmitter in your brain. Turkey is a high source of tryptophan and the smell of it cooking is very soothing. It takes little extra effort to roast a few veggies with the bird. Comforting family food on a weeknight.

Ingredients

1 tbsp	grapeseed oil	heart-healthy oil
1½ lb	bone-in turkey breast	tryptophan; lifts mood
½ cup	white wine	phytonutrients
½ cup	chicken broth	flavourful lean protein
½ tsp	garlic powder	allicin; fights fungus
1 tsp	thyme leaves	chlorophyll; cleanses blood

Benefits

Preheat oven to 400°F. Warm a skillet over medium-high heat. Add grapeseed oil to the pan and place the breast in, skin side down. Sear for 2–3 minutes. Pour in wine and allow it to deglaze the pan and evaporate for 2 minutes. Turn breast over and pour in broth. Sprinkle with garlic powder and thyme and cover pan with foil. Place pan into oven and cook turkey breast through, for about 60 minutes or until internal temperature is 185°F. Remove breast and carve; serve broth as a jus.

Preparation time: 20 minutes Servings: 4 to 6

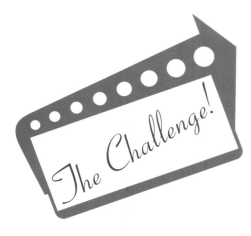

The Challenge!

LEARN TO BREATHE — properly! Most of us hold our breath and defensively tighten our shoulders. The more we do this, the less oxygen gets to our cells, and the less productive our bodies' processes are. When we feel stress, the body perceives danger and releases hormones to help us "fight or flee." These hormones cause blood pressure and heart rate to increase. When the danger turns out not to be life threatening, just a manuscript deadline or a missed doctor's appointment, we need to know how to bring our state of alarm back to normal or we will suffer the consequences of sustained stress. By actively learning to breathe we tell our stress hormones to take a hike.

1. Sit in your chair or lie on the ground with one hand on your upper chest, below the collarbone. Your other hand rests just above your navel. Your goal is to make the belly-button hand move as much as possible upward without raising the collarbone. It may take a few tries; be careful not to hyperventilate. Start with five breaths. Stop and come back to this exercise later.

2. Breathe in through your nose to the count of four, pause for as long as is comfortable, then breathe out through your mouth to the count of eight. Or, faster in, pause, and slower out. This process engages the parasympathetic nervous system, which tells the stressed-out sympathetic nervous system to slow down, rest, and relax. You want to shoot for as many deep breaths as you can in a day; I aim for at least six per hour (one every 10 minutes), but there is no magic number. I have trained myself to remember to breathe. Before I go on set, or to an interview or into a meeting that is scaring the crap out of me, I take 10 deep breaths and as a result I rarely look or feel nervous.

3. Set your watch, BlackBerry, or timer to go off once per hour during the workday this week. Do the breathing exercises described in steps 1 and 2. By the weekend, you will be automatically breathing better and you will feel much less stressed out as a result.

Now, you can more easily tackle that list of things that *are* within your control.

TEN OF DIAMONDS

THE BENEFITS OF LAUGHTER: Nothing like a good chuckle

I was a very serious kid, luckily raised by a very playful mother. Without her, I would never have learned to laugh at myself and the world around me. If I don't get a good gut-laugh every day, the day seems dreary indeed. It is usually me in a meeting (even some pretty serious ones) who bravely cracks the first joke. Everyone appreciates the levity and you can almost feel the stress in the room go down and the meeting instantly become more productive.

Some of the funniest men I have ever known were a group of homicide detectives that I had the pleasure of working with in a previous career in the hotel business. They performed one of the most difficult and least funny jobs going, and humour was their key coping mechanism.

There are loads of studies showing that laughter can reduce stress. Stress can be measured by checking markers like blood pressure and cortisol (a stress hormone) levels before and after laughter. Other studies reveal that laughter is associated with reduced perception of pain. There is also evidence that endorphins and immune cells increase and muscles relax with the physical and emotional release of laughter, which is free and painless and has no negative side effects.

One interesting study reported that people with heart disease tended to have personalities that responded with less humour to everyday situations. This conclusion led researchers to believe that learning to laugh more often can be cardioprotective. Chemical analysis has shown that the tears released when you have dust or onion in your eyes is different from the tears due to grief or joy. Even if they are tears of sadness, the release leaves you calmer and grateful for the moment. And there is nothing like the feeling of laughing so hard that you cry!

The proponents of laughter therapy would have you believe that it cures cancer and the naysayers would have you believe that the studies are biased. Who cares? The bottom line is that laughter makes you feel good and it makes the others around you feel even better. It is socially contagious — as anyone who frequents comedy clubs or funny movies will tell you. On top of it all, if you ask just about any woman what attracts her to her man, she will likely say, "He makes me laugh." So the trick is to cultivate a life that helps you laugh. If you are not a natural laugher, you may have to work a little harder. If you are a laugher, your game will be to see how often or hard you can laugh.

Here are some ways of increasing your laughter quotient:

- Hang out with funny friends.
- Don't be afraid to *be* a funny friend.
- Find the co-workers who will chuckle with you rather than gripe.
- Find ways to bump up the humour in every situation.
- Look for the irony in every circumstance.
- Go to comedies or comedy clubs.
- Search out a laughter group, people who gather just for the sake of laughing together. It may seem contrived but many swear by the results!
- Act like a 13-year-old and look for funny, random video clips on YouTube.
- If you feel it coming on, let 'er rip! My mother always said: "It's worse to stifle a laugh than a sneeze."

MY JOKE OF THE WEEK!

There once was a wise guy named Artie, who, back in 1920, was paid $1 to kill a competing grocer suspected of trying to muscle in on a family's business. Artie snuck into the grocer's store early in the morning when he figured there would be no witnesses and got the job done. When he turned to see that there were two witnesses, he felt he had to finish the job and took care of them as well.
The headline in the evening paper was: "Artie Chokes 3 for a Dollar!"

SIMMERED ARTICHOKES

If this is your first time eating artichokes, you'll need a couple of pointers. The edible portion of the leaves is the base. Pull one leaf off at a time and scrape the inside of it on your bottom teeth. When you get to the centre (heart), you will find a soft, fleshy core that is intended to be eaten whole.

	Ingredients	*Benefits*
½ tsp	sea salt	trace minerals
1 tsp	lemon juice	cleanses kidneys
3	artichokes	lower cholesterol
2 tbsp	butter	protects essential fatty acids in our cells
½ tsp	herbes de Provence	multiple-source micronutrients
1	garlic clove, minced	boosts immunity

Bring a large pot of water to a boil and add sea salt. Fill a large bowl with cold water and add lemon. Cut one artichoke in half from stem to tip and use a spoon to scoop out the core where the fibrous hairs are and discard it. Immediately plunge artichoke half into lemon water to prevent browning and continue process with remaining artichokes.

Lift artichokes with a slotted spoon from cold water into boiling water. Stir occasionally. Boil uncovered for 10–15 minutes, depending upon the size of artichokes. The heart, at the base of the vegetable, should be soft enough to poke with a fork. Drain. Set artichokes cut side up on a platter.

Melt butter in a small dish in the microwave. Stir in herbes de Provence and garlic and pour over artichokes. If you are making ahead, this dish can be stored and baked at 350°F for 10 minutes to reheat. (Pouring a fixed amount of butter as opposed to dipping leaves reduces the amount of fat you are likely to consume.)

Preparation time: 15 minutes Servings: 2 to 4

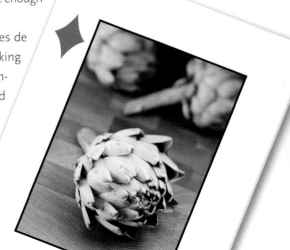

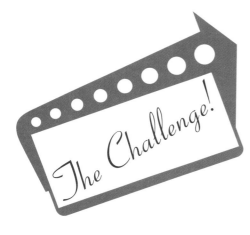

The Challenge!

WRITE DOWN TEN THINGS that tickle your funny bone, that make you laugh or even chuckle. For me, it's physical comedy. Just picturing a Jack Tripper moment makes me chortle. I bet you'll smile just writing them down.

1. _____

2. _____

3. _____

4. _____

5. _____

6. _____

7. _____

8. _____

9. _____

10. _____

NINE OF DIAMONDS

SWEAT: Maybe we *should* sweat the small stuff?

Skin is the largest organ in the body, and among its many jobs (beyond keeping your guts inside) is to eliminate waste through our pores. Sweat, which is composed mostly of water, gets rid of normal bodily wastes, like uric acid, and of excess trace minerals (potassium, calcium, magnesium, zinc, copper), and of unwanted heavy metals, like lead and aluminum. There are two types of sweat: eccrine and apocrine.

We generate eccrine sweat through all of our pores from birth; it regulates temperature and removes wastes. At puberty we develop apocrine glands in the armpit and groin areas. These glands release a waxy sweat in response to emotions like stress or arousal and pheromones to attract potential mates. Neither type of sweat stinks unless bacteria stay too close to the body for too long. We sweat out an average of about two cups per day before we even factor in heat or exercise.

Now that you know that skin is very active you need to maximize its efforts in two ways: sweat more for better elimination of waste products and work in the opposite direction by absorbing a crucial element, magnesium. In order to increase sweating we need to raise the body's temperature through exercise and heat. When

you generate sweat during exertion your body's job is to move water through the skin to cool you off and keep your cells' electrolytes in balance. This kind of sweating expels mainly the excess trace minerals your body accumulates.

The heated environment of a steam bath, sauna, or induction sauna helps increase the elimination of heavy metals, which takes pressure off the work that your kidneys and bladder have to do. It also increases circulation without exertion, which is beneficial to people who are unable to exercise. It raises the heart rate and brings blood to the surface of the skin, giving even the tiniest capillaries a workout. The relaxation that results is a precious bonus. Allowing body temperature to rise and then return to normal has been shown to ease aches and pains of everyone from athletes to those suffering from arthritis and fibromyalgia. In short, do sweat the small stuff.

Your skin not only eliminates outward; it also absorbs inward. Soaking in Epsom salts is a time-honoured way to relax after a good hike, ski, or chopping down a tree. Epsom salts are primarily magnesium. The Queen of Hearts began to explain the role of this necessary mineral in helping the body sleep. Magnesium factors in to your body's ability to balance its fluids, create enzymes (which are needed for every process in the human body), control muscles (including the heart), produce energy, lower blood pressure, improve the use of insulin, and bind serotonin (for the feel-good messages in the brain). That's a pretty powerful little mineral.

It is estimated that North Americans' magnesium levels have dropped more than 50 percent in the last century, partly because our food supply and monoculture growing methods have depleted our soils but also because we are not choosing enough of the magnesium-rich foods like whole grains, fruits, nuts, and seeds. Bathing in Epsom salts is an easy way to replenish. Studies show that blood levels of magnesium increase when we soak in a bath of at least 50°F with a concentration of an average tub of water and about two cups of Epsom salts. Doing so two to three times per week can raise the magnesium in your blood to protective levels.

Combining sweating out effectively with absorbing inwardly is a one-two punch. A weekly sauna or steam bath and a couple of soaks in Epsom salts will do the trick.

STEAMED SALMON WITH SNOW PEAS

Steaming is an ancient, low-fat way to quickly cook food and a
$9 bamboo steamer basket is all you need.

Ingredients

		Benefits
1	leek, chopped	manganese for bone density
1½ cups	white wine	tyrosol; protects against cell oxidation
½	juice of lemon	alkalizing when digested
2 lb	salmon fillets	protein for cell structure
1 tbsp	dill	eugenol; helps control blood sugar
4 cups	snow peas	vitamin K1, helps build bone
1 tbsp	fresh lemon zest	potent phytonutrients
1 tbsp	butter	thickens sauce without cream
	sea salt to taste	minerals for bone density

Trim leek and rinse well under running water. Chop white part and set aside to include in the steaming water. Lay a few of the dark leaves in bottom of a steamer basket to prevent fish from sticking.

Add wine, lemon juice and chopped leek to a large pot filled with water and bring to a boil over high heat. Place salmon in steamer basket on top of leek leaves. Set over steam and cover. Cook for 6–8 minutes or until fish is opaque throughout. (This step very much depends upon the size and thickness of your fish, so be sure to check that there is enough water to get the job done without boiling dry; top up if needed.) While fish is cooking, rinse and trim dill, rinse snow peas, and zest a lemon.

When fish is cooked, remove to a platter. Add butter to remaining liquid (if it has all evaporated, add ¼ cup of wine). Add snow peas to wine and leek sauce. Cover and cook for 1 minute. Pour snow peas and sauce over fish and serve immediately topped with dill, lemon zest, and sea salt.

Preparation time: 10 minutes Serves: 6

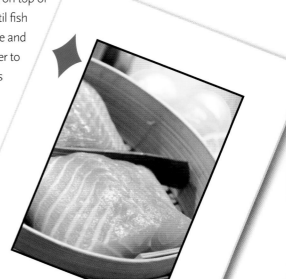

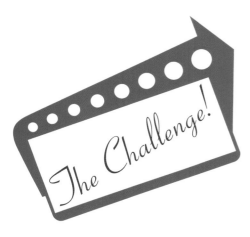

The Challenge!

FIND A WAY TO sweat it out. A friend with a sauna is a friend indeed, but your local Y or community or fitness centre may have a sauna or steam room. If possible, buy a pass of at least four visits and go once a week for a month. If you belong to a gym or club that has a steam room or sauna, ask if you can bring a friend or family member in for a "hot time," or encourage the management to sell family passes to these facilities.

EIGHT OF DIAMONDS

H2O: Eight glasses a day? Really?

When I was growing up, people said, "You must drink eight glasses of water per day." Then I heard, "It has to be pure water, not juice or tea." Lately, the cry has been, "You must have eight glasses of water per day *and* it has to be pure water, not juice or tea, *and* you can't count on your sensation of thirst; you are dehydrated before you feel it." Hold on a minute! Not only are these dictums getting longer, they are also becoming more complicated and difficult. Don't we have enough to feel guilty about?

It is true that many of us are chronically dehydrated, partly due to our high salt intake and our low fruit and vegetable intake. You will find evidence to support either position: eight glasses per day or drink when you are thirsty. But your hydration needs depend on a myriad of factors:

- your size, shape, and gender
- the number of pores you have (who's counting those?)
- the amount that you sweat
- your day-to-day stress levels
- your genetics
- the environment that you live in (hot and dry? cold and wet? heated or air conditioned?)
- the amount of high-water-content foods that you eat (*Ace Your Health* has changed this already!)
- your caffeine and alcohol intake
- your medications

Consider all of these factors when figuring out how much water you should be drinking and, most importantly, listen to what your body tells you. Some signs of even minor dehydration are:

- dry mouth
- dry skin
- dry hair and nails
- headaches
- light-headedness
- constipation

But the best way to figure out if you are consuming enough liquid is to monitor the colour of your urine. Your goal each day is clear, colourless pee.

In the morning, your urine may be artificially yellow or fluorescent green from supplements you are taking, but if you drink enough water it will turn clear before the end of the day.

The Nine of Diamonds showed how important it is to sweat, but you also need to replace that output. Remember that fruits, vegetables, and herbal and low-caffeine teas (like green and white) do contribute to your water intake. They also bring with them a raft of nutrients and few calories.

Staying hydrated is a great way to help you control your weight. It is easy to confuse the thirst signal with the hunger signal, and if you drink a glass of water before giving in to your cravings you may find it helps you resist. Green tea is an even better appetite suppressant. When you see or smell a food (or even think of a food) that you are craving, your salivary glands start producing digestive enzymes in your mouth to help digest that food. Green tea changes that chemistry immediately, which may turn off that "feed me!" alarm going off in your brain. Boost your willpower by drinking a cup of green tea (even decaf) before indulging in something sinful next time.

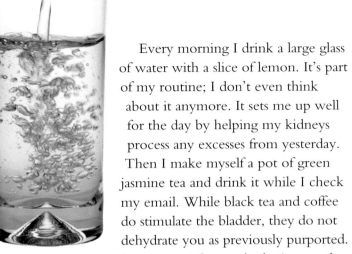

Every morning I drink a large glass of water with a slice of lemon. It's part of my routine; I don't even think about it anymore. It sets me up well for the day by helping my kidneys process any excesses from yesterday. Then I make myself a pot of green jasmine tea and drink it while I check my email. While black tea and coffee do stimulate the bladder, they do not dehydrate you as previously purported. They may not be as rehydrating as other liquids but they don't dehydrate *as long as you are also drinking other liquids*.

The downside of juices and sugary beverages is that they add (often empty) calories to a cup that should be calorie-free. We didn't evolve to drink caloric liquids – there were no juicers in the cave! Whole fruits bring some earth-infused (and therefore nutrient-rich) liquid with them.

Your goal is to find a pleasurable way to increase your amount of calorie-free liquids like water and herbal tea. If they don't have sugar, artificial sweeteners, or caffeine attached to them, even better.

WATERMELON SLUSHIE

Slushies are based on *granita*, a peasant version of ice cream. It is basically frozen fruit that is high in water and natural sugar and is granular when frozen. Adding wine keeps the slushie from freezing completely. This is an easy, no-bake dessert that goes well with dark chocolate at the end of a fancy or simple meal.

Ingredients

		Benefits
4–5 cups	seedless watermelon	
	(1 mini watermelon)	beta carotene; protects eyes
3 cups	dessert wine, brandy, or ice wine	
	(with at least 17% alcohol to	
	prevent water from freezing)	tyrosol; protects heart cells

Scoop flesh and juice of watermelon into a blender and pulse until liquid. Add wine, pulse until blended. Pour into a pretty, shallow bowl and place into the freezer for at least 6 hours. Use a fork to scrape and loosen the crystals for easier serving.

Preparation time: 6 to 8 minutes Servings: 12 to 16

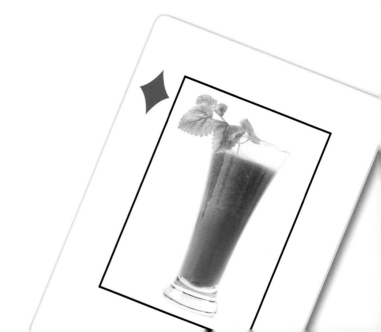

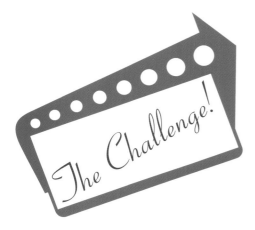

FIND THE MOST BEAUTIFUL glass bottle of fancy water in your local supermarket or health food store. It should hold 750 millilitres or one litre. Don't worry about what is inside, or where it comes from. Pour the contents into a glass and drink over the course of the day. Every morning after, fill that bottle with clean, clear, filtered tap water and set it in a place where you will see it all day long. Pour small amounts into a glass or cup and sip throughout the day. Do this each and every day from here on in. It costs little to nothing, takes no time, is visually pleasing, and is a positive habit that keeps you healthily hydrated.

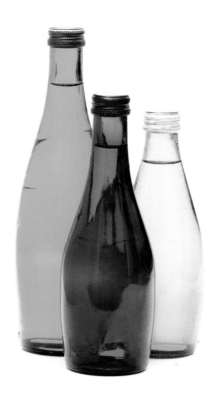

SEVEN OF DIAMONDS

HEALTHY HEARING:
If a bird sings in the city, does anybody hear it?

———————

The definition of a weed is a plant growing in an unwanted place. This leaves a lot open to interpretation. For instance, I have wild mint growing in the crevices of my front garden. While others may consider this a weed and pull it out, I like it because it covers some ugly rock and blooms a beautiful blue.

The same goes with noise. What might be a beautiful sound to some could easily be considered an intrusive noise by others. I grew up living near a major highway, while my husband grew up next to the ocean. Luckily, both make the same *shhhhhhh shhhhhhh shhhhhh* sound and feel like soothing white noise to us. I love the buzz of a Manhattan sidewalk, but the honking makes me jumpy. The sound of crickets or cicadas on a summer night in the country is like a symphony to me but an annoyance to others. It is all about perspective.

There is sound (ha!) evidence that the more intrusive sounds of a jackhammer, airplane, car horn, alarm, or barking dog have a negative impact upon our health. Unwanted loud noise causes stress, which can be measured through the increase of stress hormones in the blood

and rising blood pressure. This is true whether you are awake or asleep, but may be even worse when asleep since the all-important, restorative REM phase may be interrupted. Noisy environments have also been shown to negatively affect concentration levels and test scores.

Hearing impairment can result from prolonged exposure to noise. Any hearing loss that I encounter was probably caused by all the rock concerts I went to in my youth, but any hearing loss my daughter and her peers experience will probably come from the ever-present earphones they wear.

For urban or suburban dwellers, much of the day is spent consciously or unconsciously blocking out noise. We don't even notice it sometimes until we are irritated and try to figure out why. And the best way to manage it is to tune in, rather than out. Noticing the sounds around you puts you back in control. As I am writing this, there is a large backhoe outside my window, digging up the street. I'm sure it's there for some important reason, but the sound is grating on my nerves. I can choose either to let it grate on me or to do something about it. Fruitlessly yelling at the driver to shut the heck up may make me feel better for a moment and release some stress, but he isn't going to stop until his job is done, and I'd rather not just pass along my irritation. Better for me to take a deep breath, notice the sound and then let it go, knowing that it will end. I could turn on some music that will cheer me up but not intrude on my work. I could turn on a fan that will mimic the sound of the beach I am imagining in my head. I could take a break and go for a walk and listen to the birds in the trees. The point is that some things are within my control and others aren't. Knowing which is which alleviates stress and anxiety.

CARAMELIZED ONIONS

There is nothing like the sound of onions frying in a pan – the sizzle and sputter as they hit the skillet and then the beehive-like hum as they simmer. The wafting smell isn't half bad either. You can use these caramelized onions in many recipes.

	Ingredients	*Benefits*
2 lb	yellow onions	Quercetin; prevents cholesterol oxidation
2 tbsp	butter	healthy saturated fat
1 tbsp	grapeseed oil	heart-healthy fat
1 tbsp	honey or maple syrup	low glycemic index sweetener
pinch	sea salt	trace minerals

Heat a cast iron skillet over medium-high heat. Roughly chop onions. Add butter and oil to the pan and add handfuls of onions, allowing each handful to cook down a little before adding more. Once all are in and softened, add honey or maple syrup and sea salt. Allow to cook over low heat, stirring often, for up to 1 hour. Store in small containers in the freezer until ready to use.

Ways to use:
- Stir into pasta with leftover chicken and parsley.
- Use to top a frittata.
- Awesome on a fried egg sandwich.
- Great soup or sauce starter.
- Add flavour to a slow-cooker meal, without salt.
- Slather on fish or chicken and bake.
- Spread on whole-wheat pizza crust and top with cheese.

Preparation time: **30 minutes** Servings: **20**

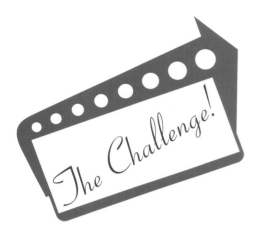

THINK ABOUT A SOUND that soothes you. For me, it's the sound of a schoolyard full of kids playing, and I will often time my breaks to take a walk past the local school during recess. Letting that sound wash over me gives great pleasure as it brings back my own happy times in grade school and my daughter's younger years. For you, it could be waves (which can be replicated by a sound machine or a blowing fan) or the bell on an ice cream truck (Google to find the sound online). This week spend two minutes every day tuning in to the sounds around you and deciding whether you like them or not. If no, a few deep breaths and a conscious decision to let your irritation go or to mask the sound is all you need. If yes, find a way to work that sound into your life and write it down here:

Sounds I like:

_____

_____

_____

_____

_____

How I will work them into my life:

_____

_____

_____

_____

_____

SIX OF DIAMONDS

SNACKS vs. TREATS: It's okay to go nuts over snacks

Let's define snacks. Snacks are *foods* that you eat daily between meals that nourish you for a few hours. Treats are less nutritious pleasure-giving foods that you should consume only weekly or monthly.

Snacks		Treats
handful of nuts		chocolate-covered almonds
2 squares of 70% dark chocolate		chocolate bars purchased at the checkout counter
small whole-grain muffin		cinnamon raisin bagel
fruit		fruit roll-ups
celery sticks		deep-fried zucchini sticks

How often do you grab a treat and call it a snack? If you add up the calories of all the treats eaten as snacks, they will outweigh the snacks by about 100 to 125 calories. Do this for a month and you have just added a pound to your body weight without even thinking about it. I wouldn't mind that pound if it was building a better brain as snacking on nuts would, or reducing inflammation as dark chocolate can, or fighting off cancer as the berries do. But for just doing nothing? Nothing gets that kind of free ride in my life!

The argument for snacking between meals is that it takes the edge off hunger, which can help you make better decisions about what to have for lunch and dinner. The benefit of a slow-burning, high-fibre, high-protein snack is that it gives your pancreas a rest. Asking your pancreas to produce moderate amounts of insulin to digest useable, useful fuel is a good bargain. Pounding it with pudding over and over again makes it rebel, which causes your stress hormones to go wild. When your pancreas rebels, you feel tired. Do this too often and your pancreas says, "I don't think so. I give up," and then you join the growing line of diabetics and pre-diabetics.

You need to have healthy snacks at hand when that hand is ready to grab food. The best snack on the planet is a handful of nuts. Anyone who lived through the 1980s is thinking, "But nuts are so high in fat!" Yes, they are. And that is why I said a handful. The good fats provide lubrication for the brain and joints, they make skin glow and hair shine, and we just don't get enough of them. But which nuts? How much? How often?

All nuts have their own nutritional profiles. Mixing a few different types makes for a nice surprise with each mouthful, and you are sure to get the many minerals they offer if you mix them up a bit. For instance, selenium is a potent nutrient that is proving to be a powerful cancer fighter. Foods grown in selenium-rich soil contain lots of the mighty mineral; foods grown in depleted soils (as in most of North America) contain little. Brazil has extraordinarily high amounts of selenium in its soil and Brazil nuts grown in this soil contain a perfect, useable form. In fact, one Brazil nut gives you all the selenium you need for the entire day.

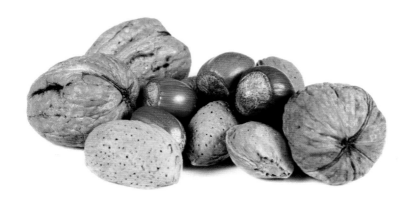

SNACK NUT MIX

You can make this recipe on the weekend and keep it in your desk drawer all week. Feel free to indulge lightly and daily. Alternating raw and salted nuts with a little something sweet hits all the right notes to satisfy any snack craving. Vary the nuts and get all the nutrients available from each.

	Ingredients	*Benefits*
1 cup	Brazil nuts	selenium for cancer prevention
1 cup	raw almonds	calcium; builds strong teeth
1 cup	salted sunflower seeds	vitamin E; anti-aging
1 cup	pumpkin seeds	low-cal omega-3 for prostate health
¼ cup	dried currants	high-antioxidant fruit

Mix all the ingredients together and store in a glass container that you can see. Have 1 small handful once per day. The combinations of nuts available are endless. Try cashews, walnuts, peanuts . . . Other berries you could use: acai berries, raisins, dried blueberries, dried cranberries (be sure all dried fruit is unsweetened).

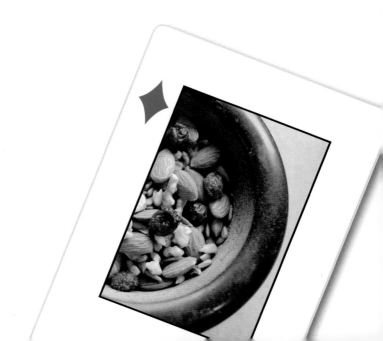

Preparation time: **2 minutes** Servings: **12**

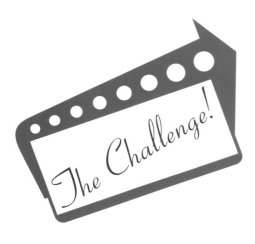

The Challenge!

THIS WEEK KEEP TRACK of your snacks versus treats. You will know it's a true snack if you can put an entry in the nutritional value column.

FOOD ITEM	NUTRITIONAL VALUE	SNACK OR TREAT?
ALMONDS	GOOD FATS/CALCIUM	S
TEA BISCUIT		T

FIVE OF DIAMONDS

FAMILY HOLIDAY EATS: Top of the list: guilt-free meals

The only way to get through holidays without blowing all your hard work is to plan ahead. Holidays bring families and friends together to celebrate and also bring out our most self-destructive habits. We learned about the social contagion of attitude on health in the Four of Spades. Knowing that our behaviour has such a powerful effect on our loved ones means we must choose to make it positive.

Many of the traditional holidays roll out in a similar way. It's usually about family and friends gathering, sitting and chatting, nibbling and drinking, eating a large meal, sitting some more, then packing in dessert. Consider this: what would happen if we planned ahead to include a walk with the kids to the park as part of the holiday activities? Maybe even a hike or a ski or a trip to apple-picking farm, or a family touch football game. There are loads of options that can be built right in and they would mean more activity and less sedentary snacking. What would happen if you offered to bring veggies and low-fat dip for the pre-dinner munching? You would effect a positive change for everyone and save yourself as many as 1,000 extra calories to work off next week. Make a conscious decision to bring a delicious vegetable side dish to replace butter- and cream-laden mashed potatoes. Helping yourself while helping the entire group is a persuasive loving act.

Let's take a look at the main course to see where we can create healthy eating strategies. Of course, Aunt Jeannie's stuffing is the best in the world, but consuming more than one tablespoon doesn't make it taste any better, and it will be there next year. The point is, we need to approach these holidays not like it is the last time we will ever eat these foods but with the belief that if we eat less of these foods we will get to enjoy them for longer.

Like any gambler, you need to know your limit *before* you begin the game. Before you even get to the party, there is a lot you can do to plan ahead and make sure that the previous week is very, very lean and full of veggies, which will allow you to accommodate the event more easily. An extra 5 to 10 minutes added daily to your cardio routine for one week can burn off 50 to 75 extra calories per day, which could free you up to eat a guilt-free piece of pie.

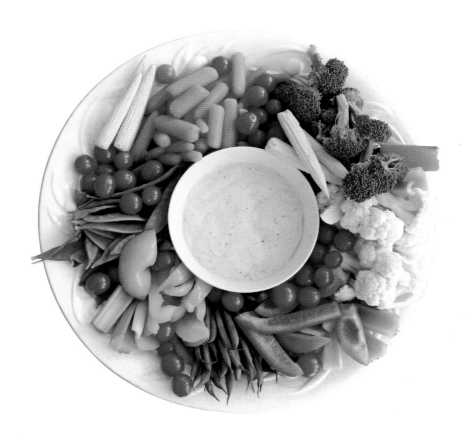

HALF-BAKED SQUASH

I called this recipe "half baked" as a bit of tongue in cheek because it wasn't all that thought out. It really was one of those "what can I toss together" kind of dishes. Feel free to mix it up any which way you would like. Any fruit adds fibre, any cheese adds flavour, and any nut adds fun. On occasion, when I have a vegetarian over, I load it up as a main course for them.

Ingredients		*Benefits*
2	small acorn squash	carotenoids; protect vision
2	small Granny Smith apples	soluble fibre; lowers cholesterol
2 tbsp	crumbled blue cheese	strong flavour means less cheese
2 tbsp	chopped walnuts	good fats for healthy joints
½ tsp	honey	phytochemicals for overall health
	black pepper, to taste	aids digestion

Wash skin and cut each squash into six wedges vertically, through the stem to tip. Scoop out seeds and discard. Microwave wedges uncovered in a casserole dish for 5–6 minutes, just to soften. Slice and core apples. In a large bowl, mix together apples, crumbled blue cheese, chopped walnuts, honey, and black pepper. Place squash wedges in a large baking dish with cut sides up and scoop filling into squash. Bake in oven at 400°F uncovered for 20–30 minutes, until squash is soft and cheese is melted.

Preparation time: **10 minutes** Servings: 6

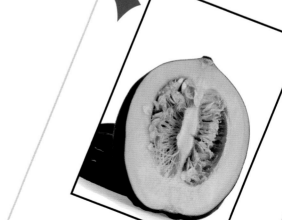

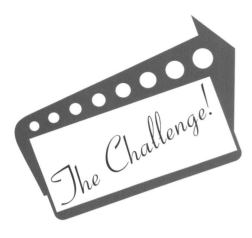
The Challenge!

WHETHER IT'S CHRISTMAS, EASTER, Thanksgiving, Chanukah, or any other "let's eat" occasion, when the big day comes, here is the game plan: visually divide the dinner plate down the middle. There will be two categories, green/steamed vegetables and lean proteins vs starchy and or/buttery vegetables and carbohydrates. You can have it all! But! Load up your plate with as much of one as you wish, the other category has to be measured. Guess which is which?! If you have one full plate of steamed green vegetables or raw salad greens before you start with the heavier stuff, you will find it easier to control your fork.

Green Vegetables and lean proteins	Starchy/buttery vegetables and Carbohydrates
Start with a plate of green then add a reasonable amount of protein (the size of your palm)	No more than a tablespoon or two of: • Mashed squash • Mashed potatoes • Buttered carrots • Stuffing • Any "casserole" type dish • Gravy • Cheese sauce • Salad dressing • Dessert

FOUR OF DIAMONDS

DESSERT: Mother, may I?

We all love a little something sweet once in a while. Let's face it, life's short, so let's enjoy it. At this stage in the game, you probably have made so many improvements, have dropped a few pounds, feel better overall, have more energy, and are wondering: "Where's the cake?"

One of the more interesting qualities that humans have is their sense of entitlement. We've all heard the little voice in our heads that says, "Come on, I've behaved all day!" and "I've worked really hard, so where's my reward?" Advertisers and marketers count on you thinking these very thoughts. The upside is that the thoughts are true: we *do* deserve treats. The downside is that they can grow into an inflated sense of entitlement, which could be our undoing.

Dessert used to be something that was served only on Sunday nights after the family meal. It was a pie baked with real whole fruit or a crumble topped with oats and butter. Taking a small slice ensured that there was enough to go around, plus you would burn off the calories doing physical activity the next day. Dessert nowadays seems to be a nightly or even twice-daily thing. The

portions are huge, as we expect to get our money's worth. Some of the seemingly innocuous cookies sold at the coffee shop contain enough fat and calories to blow an entire day of wise choices and yet we are eating them with our coffee, as breakfast or an afternoon snack. And we may still feel a little cheated if we don't get something sweet after dinner.

It's important to know that our taste buds only perceive the acute sweetness of the first few bites of a dessert. After that, it is mindless motion intended to finish the plate. This is a part of the reason that French women don't get fat. They expect better quality and accept smaller portion sizes.

If you want to keep your calorie count in check, you can indulge in dessert maybe once per week. Make sure that you choose something that you love, then sit down with someone whom you love and share it. Or have it in the middle of the afternoon with a cup of tea so that you can truly experience and enjoy it. Dessert after a meal is often just a waste; you stuff it in because you can, not because your body needs it. I have challenged many a fellow diner to tell me that they truly enjoyed the richness of dessert at the end of a big meal. Three bites is really all anyone has ever admitted to appreciating.

If you have a sweet tooth and just can't seem to break the nightly habit, try storing a variety of sugarless gum right next to the sweets drawer, and instead of indulging pop a stick of gum in your mouth. It may not work every night, but if you can do so every other night, you are making progress. Or keep some hard candies made from maple sugar and suck on one when you get a craving for something sweet. Candies create saliva and satisfy the "sweeten me" signal easily. Even better, switch up your multivitamin with a kids' chewable version. Many vitamins and supplements come in chewable formats: omega-3s, vitamin C, zinc. You could have yourself a nice little treat of chewy candy that is really working for you instead of 500 calories' worth of ice cream that will only let you down.

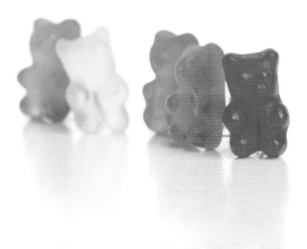

DATE SQUARES

I love date squares and luckily they aren't unhealthy, just caloric. But when the calories come from such powerful ingredients, I am happy to choose this dessert often.

Ingredients / *Benefits*

FILLING:

3 cups	pitted dates	high in potassium; lowers blood pressure
1 tbsp	orange zest	potent antioxidants
1½ tbsp	unsalted butter	zero impact on cholesterol levels
1 cup	water	

CRUMBLE:

2½ cups	rolled oats	magnesium and fibre; lower blood pressure
1¼ cups	whole-wheat flour, or spelt	fibre for regularity
½ cup	maple syrup	high-mineral sweetener
1 tbsp	cinnamon	controls blood sugar
⅔ cup	salted butter, melted	good fat; protects vision

Preheat oven to 350°F. Place all the filling ingredients into a pot and boil for 3–5 minutes. Mash with a fork or potato masher to a thick purée. Let stand uncovered. Line an 8-inch-square baking pan with parchment paper. In a large bowl, mix oats, flour, maple syrup, and cinnamon. Melt butter and stir into crumble. Press half of crumble very firmly into lined pan and top with date mixture. Top with remaining crumble, but do not press. Bake uncovered for 45–50 minutes. Cool in fridge before serving. Cut into 16 squares.

Preparation time: 15 minutes Servings: 16

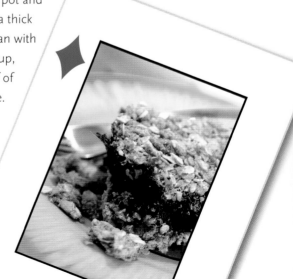

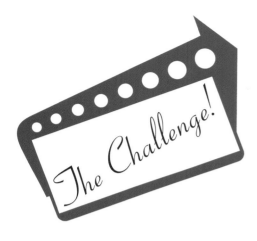
The Challenge!

COMMIT TO DECIDING. BY that I mean, rather than simply consuming dessert, actually make a decision that you want it. Decide before it touches your lips how many mouthfuls you will have and remove the remainder to another plate, container, or a friend's plate. If you *really, really* love something, you should have it, and you are right to feel entitled. For instance, there is no way I can go to Quebec without having **tarte au sucre** (the equivalent of pecan pie without the pecans – and way better). Luckily I am in that province only occasionally. I let myself make a game out of sussing out the best **tarte** by savouring small amounts of all available options rather than fully consuming every one. This way, I don't feel deprived, but I have only had one or two bites of the less stellar versions and have kept my eye on the prize of the perfect **tarte**.

My favourite dessert is: _____.

The best one I ever ate was at _____.

Commit to remaining true to that standard and enjoying your fave (even up to once a week) fully.

THREE OF DIAMONDS

THE PLANET: What's that got to do with my health?

No doubt by now you've noticed that I've sprinkled in a little earth awareness here and there throughout this book. The truth is that I try to see my life through green-tinted glasses. Once I got the hang of it, it wasn't hard to give up caustic scouring powders in favour of baking soda, or pine-smelly disinfectants for vinegar, and I saved a few dollars to boot. With each and every purchasing decision I make, I try to factor in whether or not this product is good – or at least less bad – for the planet. (The fact that I am inhaling less toxic stuff is a side benefit.) There is no excuse these days for not seeking out green alternatives; all of the large manufacturers are jumping on the bandwagon and making huge leaps in their products.

But to be honest, I am really "going green" for selfish reasons. The impact of caring for the planet is connected to my health in several ways:

- Everything comes back to earth eventually: fuel emissions, pesticides, toxic chemicals, etc.
- Riding my Vespa to work makes me feel young, saves money on gas and parking, and takes up less space in city traffic.
- Avoiding toxic chemicals keeps me healthy longer, which costs us all less in the long run.

We are a one-car family that uses public transit, a scooter, or bicycles most of the time.

The next vehicle we buy will be a hybrid because there are now vehicles in the size category that we need that are within our financial reach. It isn't just the emissions that I am eliminating during my errand runs (though the benefits definitely start there); it is also the noise. Hybrid vehicles are quieter, so they have less noise pollution impact in my neighbourhood. This means that I am not revving up my neighbours' nerves any more than need be each time I zoom around the block (see Seven of Diamonds). But the key benefit is that the peaceful ride reduces my stress. I feel more at ease in the silence, which in turn has an impact on my family (if I am less stressed, I am less crabby and more productive). If their days go better as a result then we have three people out in the world giving all they have got *and* causing fewer emissions.

The list of harmful things that I want to reduce or eliminate starts with:

- pesticides on food
- toxic cleansers in water
- parabens and phthalates in skin care products
- vehicle emissions
- the amount of energy used to power computers and other electronic devices

I try to make a small shift in each and every category. I buy organic when I can, use baking soda, vinegar, borax, and low-surfactant laundry soap for washing up, buy unscented skin care stuff, and purchase energy from a green-energy supplier, Bullfrog Power, for our home. A few of these items cost a bit more but most actually cost less in the long run. As consumers, we do have options, and the good ones are only a decision away.

But my efforts aren't just for the planet; it all comes back to my well-being and that of the people I love. My car idling in summer city traffic has a direct impact on my asthmatic mother's ability to take a walk. My toilet bowl cleanser goes into Lake Ontario, harming the plants and the fish that live in there. I drink filtered tap water but that filter can't remove every molecule of unwanted chemicals or medications from my glass. Only we can do that by not putting them in there in the first place. If reducing the amount of stuff I slather on my face, hair, and skin, or using a cast iron skillet over a non-stick pan, means less likelihood of cancer (and it does), then I may not have taken up a hospital bed and resources to treat another needless illness. These small actions can help to reduce everyone's burden.

BREAKFAST FRUIT CRUMBLE

Two of the most affordable and readily available organic foods are apples and rolled oats. They go almost head to head with non-organic on price, making the decision an easy one. Baking an entire pan of breakfast crumble early in the week saves time, and uses less energy than heating up a frying pan daily. Hemp seeds grow readily without pesticides and replenish the soil with nitrogen, while most other crops only deplete it. In this one recipe, you can create four benefits to the planet. See how easy it is?

Ingredients		*Benefits*
¼ cup	butter, softened	easily digested
4	organic apples, unpeeled	fibre; lowers cholesterol
¾ cup	organic rolled oats	beta-glucan fibres; curb appetite
¼ cup	organic cane sugar	trace minerals and fibre
¼ cup	organic whole-wheat flour	less processing, cleaner earth
¼ cup	hemp seeds	pesticide free
1 tsp	cinnamon	high ORAC score
1 tsp	nutmeg	relieves nausea
¼ cup	water	hydrating

Preheat oven to 375°F. Put butter into a 9-inch square pan and place in oven until butter melts. Wash and slice apples. When butter is melted, spread it evenly around bottom of pan and stir in oats, cane sugar, flour, hemp seeds, cinnamon, and nutmeg. Mix well. Toss in apples and be sure to mix crumble well throughout. Pour water over top. Bake 35 minutes. Serve with ½ cup organic, plain, non-fat yogurt or non-fat vanilla yogurt.

Preparation time: **20 minutes** Servings: 8

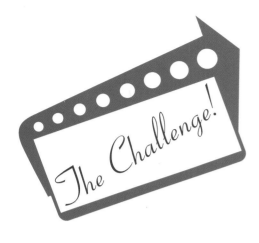

The Challenge!

WHAT CAN YOU DO to reduce your carbon and planetary footprint? Educate yourself first and then make as many small shifts as you can. You might start with one or two of these suggestions:

- Get regular updates from a green website of your choice.

- Buy a book about going green.

- Investigate the differences between green products and "regular" products.

- Find out more about green-energy source Bullfrog Power (*www.bullfrogpower.com*).

- Test-drive a hybrid just for fun and listen to the sounds of silence.

TWO OF DIAMONDS

BEING A GOOD SAMARITAN: Pay it forward

Simply put, doing good is good for you. You know that feeling you get when you drop off a casserole to a sick friend, or when you help a woman lift her child's stroller onto the bus. When you donate your time or your sound system to the school play, there it is again. It is in these little ways that we give to the world – but make no mistake, it gives us so much more back.

When you practise "random acts of kindness," you feel a little blip of positive emotion, a jumping in the belly, a tear in the eye that makes your step skip and your heart swell. The endorphin release that you obtain when you do something nice for another person is like none other. The lift, the high, can brighten your day and the other person's. Is it for this reason that we give? Of course not. But if we each embraced the idea that giving can give us back twofold, then everyone would be further ahead. And isn't that what we all want?

I want to live in a world where kindness is common and giving is a given. That world existed in the minds of great people like Gandhi, Mother Teresa, and John Lennon. Imagine. When you truly embrace your life, your day, and

your "self" with kindness and create a better world within and without, it is easy to give in ways that are big or small. People often smile at me on the street and I wonder: "What the heck is that lunatic grinning at?" And then I realize I was mulling over some pleasant private thought that made me smile. As a result, *I* am the lunatic grinning at nothing. People will smile back, you know. It is such a simple way to give to the world and I do it each and every day. And it always comes back. In spades.

I included the recipe for Begged, Borrowed, and Roasted Vegetable Soup here because it reminds me of the "Stone Soup" story. It is a folk tale told to children, in many cultures and with many variations, to illustrate the benefits of sharing. It goes something like this. Starving beggars stumble into a town and have trouble convincing any one person to feed them a meal. They fill a pot with water, place a stone in it, and hang the pot in the town square. Curious passersby are invited to flavour the soup with tiny morsels of ingredients. The eventual result is a delicious soup to which everyone has contributed. In this recipe the story is reversed. We all know someone who could use a good meal and wouldn't dream of asking: a new mom, an elderly aunt, a teacher having a tough time . . . So you gather the ingredients and pull the community together to help. Send out an email inviting friends, family, and neighbours to contribute ingredients for this roasted vegetable soup. Each and every person will feel and enjoy the benefits of collaborating and sharing and your community will be drawn closer together. Oh, the power of a simple soup!

BEGGED, BORROWED, AND ROASTED VEGETABLE SOUP

Ingredients		*Benefits*
1	yellow onion, chopped	donated
3	small zucchinis, cubed	donated
3	red bell peppers, diced	donated
3	small yellow potatoes, cubed	donated
6	fresh Italian plum tomatoes, chopped	donated
	garlic cloves, unpeeled	donated
1–2 tbsp	extra virgin olive oil	donated
1 tbsp	dried basil	donated
1 tbsp	dried rosemary	donated
4 cups	low-sodium beef or vegetable broth	donated
½ cup	grated cheese, any type	donated

Heat the oven to 400°F. Toss the vegetables and garlic cloves with oil on a very large cookie sheet. Sprinkle with basil and rosemary. Bake in the oven for 45–60 minutes, or until all the vegetables are tender. Bring broth to a simmer, squeeze roasted garlic from skins into soup, and add the vegetables. This soup is terrific chunky or, if you prefer it creamy, purée with a hand wand or blender. Deliver soup to a friend who is having a rough time. Top each bowl with cheese just before serving.

Preparation time: **20 minutes** Servings: 6

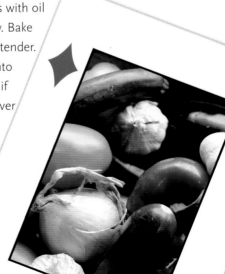

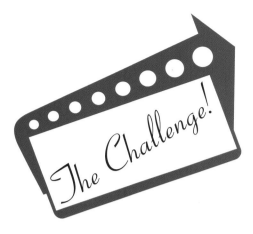

The Challenge!

CHOOSE A CHARITY. DONATE time, money, effort – whatever you can. Donate this book to someone who needs it or just give a smile to the homeless man on the corner.

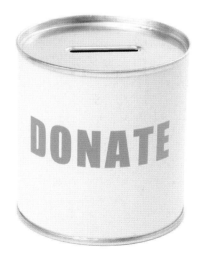

ACKNOWLEDGEMENTS

When the landscape of knowledge is constantly changing as it is in the health world it is wise to count upon the voices that one trusts. When I needed advice, guidance or specific questions answered I counted on the following people and their depth of knowledge:

Neelam Bains, Osteopath and RMT; Aileen Burford-Mason, Ph.D. immunology; Pamela Farquar, Kinesiologist/Personal Trainer; Annabel Fitsimmons, Certified Yoga and Pilates instructor; Dr. Melissa Hershberg, BSC MD CCFP; Dr. Brian Sher, D.C.; Dr. Fabio Varlese, MD, FRCPC Internal and Geriatric Medicine; Dr. Bernard Zylberberg, MD, allergist.

I also had the help of numerous recipe testers who put their own families through the purchasing, preparing and tasting of new foods and gave their comments to improve them. This group numbers in the hundreds and includes all the wise and advising women at my coffee klatch as well as my new friends on Twitter.

On the subject of my coffee klatch girls: you are like family.

This book wasn't even a twinkle in my eye until an agent called out of the blue and said "Hi, I'm Hilary McMahon with Westwood Creative Artists. What are you working on?" At the time I said "nothin.'" She unearthed my true potential, guided the project and found it a home. "Home" became McClelland & Stewart and specifically Liz Kribs who saw exactly what I wanted to do with this book and made it even better.

My production partner, Pat McGowan, and his team at InMotion are a constant source of inspiration and motivation in bringing *Ace Your Health* into the virtual realm. And, when I needed visual guidance, Mercedes Rothwell, graphic designer extraordinaire, showed the way.

My mother, Huguette Chenier, guided our health before we knew what was happening. My sisters, Michele Walker and Cheryl Mueller, are my inspiration. I keep them and their "normal" patterns of eating and excercizing behaviour firmly in mind when writing. They are more like any reader than I am and remind me all the time of what a "freak" I am with all my healthy habits.

My husband, Guy Ratchford, and our daughter, Jameson, complete the team. I'd be in any boat with these two; in stormy weather and blue skies alike I couldn't choose a tighter squad.

INDEX

PHOTO CREDITS

Dreamstime Images: Elnur Amikishiyev 231; Marilyn Barbone 217; Eugene Bochkarev 72; Sinisa Botas 187; Briancweed 50; Brybs 114; Kathy Burns-millyard 184; Cammeraydave 201; Denise Campione 113; Stephen Coburn 99; Darvidanoar 58; Dreamstock 74; Kateryna Dyellalova 103; Elena Elisseeva 28; Mark Fairey 222; Hugo Felix 245; Dmitry Fisher 132; Michael Flippo 47; Fotografieberlin 209; Stephaniefrey 27; Tracy Hebden 77; Hlphoto 176; Irochka 243; Rafa Irusta 63; Ingvald Kaldhussater 89; Kamensky 45; Simon Krzic 117; Kuleczka 57; Viktorija Kuprijanova 234; Chris Lorenz 85; Luckynick 108; Olga Lyubkina 86; Robyn Mackenzie 118; Mailthepic 129; Mike_kiev 249; Multiart61 113; Antonio Muñoz Palomares 167; Niderlander 179; Andrey Pavlov 133; Pixelbunneh 55; Pjmorley 237; Elena Ray 33; Christina Richards 241; Richardtbarnes 229; Andres Rodriguez 154; Anna Rogal 230; Guy Salah 152; Torsten Schon 87; Ferdinand Steen 100; James Steidl 137; Itay Uri 242; Stephen Vanhorn 138; Vaskoni 24; Ivonne Wierink 125; Feng Yu 255;

Author's Images: 29, 40, 80, 92, 96, 122, 134, 144, 157, 169, 172, 203, 214, 226, 238, 246, 254

MEAL PLANNER

RECIPES

Breakfast
- Magic Muesli
- Room Service Banana Oatmeal

Lunch
- Salad with Miso Dressing and Almond Chicken
- Mediterranean Lentils with a side salad
- Barbecued Chicken Wrap

Snack
- Apple Spice Muffin
- Homemade Crackers
- Iced Maple Cappuccino

Supper
- Trumped-Up 'Za
- One-Pot Tomato Sauce over whole wheat pasta
- Roast Chicken Dijon

RECIPES

Breakfast
- Dark Chocolate Shake
- Sun-dried Tomato Egg Puffs

Lunch
- Tuna or shrimp salad
- Salad with Creamy Avocado Dressing
- Serious Green Soup

Snack
- Goat Cheese and Arti-choke Spread and Crackers
- loose leaf tea
- Sleepnut Cookies

Supper
- Seafood Salsa
- Barbecued Small Fish
- Steak with Spice Rub
- Tea-Steeped Pork Tenderloin
- Creamy Yogurt Sauce on whole wheat pasta or chicken
- Cane and Able for an evening drink

♣ RECIPES

Breakfast
- Cherry Smoothie
- Cast Iron Corn Bread with walnuts
- Fruit salad with yogurt

Lunch
- Wilted Wild Green Salad with protein
- Dorowat with salad
- Microwave Grilled Chicken with salad

Snack
- Taramasalata
- Best Popcorn Ever
- Spiced Nuts
- ORAC Hot Cocoa
- Blueberry Dream

Supper
- Baby Bok Choy with Baked Tofu
- Pan-Fried Turmeric Fish
- Crab-Stuffed Crepes

RECIPES

Breakfast
- Breakfast Fruit Crumble

Lunch
- Red Lentil and Sweet Potato Soup
- Half-Baked Squash
- Begged, Borrowed, and Roasted Vegetable Soup

Snack
- Easy Focaccia
- Snack Nut Mix
- Date Square
- Watermelon Slushie

Supper
- Kiwi Salsa with baked fish
- Weeknight Turkey and Simmered Artichokes
- Steamed Salmon with Snow Peas
- Caramelized Onions in Frittata

CHALLENGE CHECKLIST

♠ Challenges:	✓
A Compare yogurt brands	
K Health store 4	
Plus new recipe	
Q Coffee counter	
J Food Court sleuth	
10 Dinner Out	
9 Convenience Brand comparison	
8 New shrimp recipe	
7 Pantry raid	
6 Bean counter	
5 Read your labels	
4 Potluck party	
3 One salad a day	
2 Drive-thru tally	

♥ Challenges:	✓
A Exercise plan	
K NEAT plan	
Q $$ magnesium	
J "Sustainable fish"	
10 Meat math	
9 Party platter avoidance	
8 Fats list	
7 Potassium foods	
6 Souped Up	
5 Saucy pal	
4 Mixology class	
3 Tea time	
2 Sock hop	

♣ Challenges:	✓
A Google "news on telomeres"	
K Vitamin D sources	
Q Go for gold	
J Fruit Salad	
10 Handfuls of Carbs	
9 Seating arrangement	
8 Sugar counter	
7 Protein Yesterday ___ tomorrow ___	
6 Egg interrogator	
5 Chicken checker	
4 Chocolate taste tester	
3 Ask an ancestor	
2 Cost of clean air	

♦ Challenges:	✓
A Choose your multivitamin	
K Find free money	
Q Stretch score	
J Learn to breathe	
10 Tickle your funny bone	
9 Sweat shop search	
8 Beautiful water bottle	
7 Sounds that soothe	
6 Snacks vs Treats	
5 Divide and measure	
4 Dessert decisions	
3 Green choice	
2 Choose a charity	